Quality Indicators

Second Edition

A Practical Guide to Assessment and Documentation

Julia Hopp, MS, RN, CNAA, BC

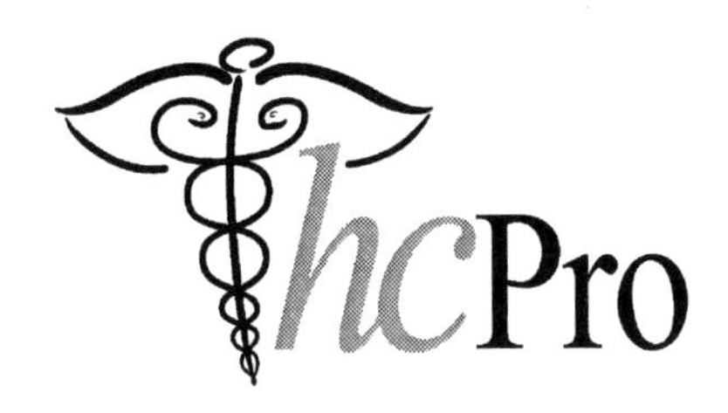

Quality Indicators, Second Edition: A Practical Guide to Assessment and Documentation is published by HCPro.

 5 4 3 2 1

ISBN 1-57839-482-1

HCPro, Inc., provides information resources for the healthcare industry.

HCPro, Inc., is not affiliated in any with the Joint Commission on Accreditation of Healthcare Organizations.

Julia Hopp, MS, RN, CNAA, BC, Author
Noelle Shough, Senior Managing Editor
Bob Croce, Group Publisher
Paul Amos, Executive Editor
Suzanne Perney, Publisher
Jean St. Pierre, Creative Director
Jackie Diehl Singer, Graphic Artist
Shane Katz, Cover Designer
Paul Singer, Layout Artist

Advice given is general. Readers should consult professional counsel for specific legal, ethical, or clinical questions.

Arrangements can be made for quantity discounts. For more information, contact:

HCPro, Inc.
P.O. Box 1168
Marblehead, MA 01945
Telephone: 800/650-6787 or 781-639-1872
Fax: 781/639-2982
E-mail: *customerservice@hcpro.com*

Visit HcPro at its World Wide Web sites:
www.hcmarketplace.com, www.hcpro.com

9/2004
20103

Contents

About the Author

Julia Hopp, MS, RN, CNAA, BC, has more than 22 years of experience in long-term care. She is currently the Vice President of Patient Accounting for the Paramount Health Care Company nursing home chain in San Antonio. Previous positions she has held include vice president of clinical services, director of reimbursement, director of nursing, nursing home administrator, and nurse consultant. Hopp is a licensed nursing home administrator and a registered nurse with an American Nurses Credentialing Center Certification in nursing administration, advanced. She has a master of science degree in health services administration from the University of St. Francis, Joliet, Il. Hopp has extensive experience in delivering presentations and seminars related to long-term care issues, Medicare and Medicaid reimbursement, and quality indicators. She is the author of the book *Long-Term Care Training Made Easy*, the senior advisor for the newsletter ***PPS Alert for Long-Term Care,*** as well as the author of the monthly question and answer column for that publication.

Acknowledgments

I would like to acknowledge HCPro, Inc., for allowing me the opportunity to pursue this topic and providing me with extensive support throughout the writing and editing process. I wish to thank Noelle Shough, senior managing editor, for her valuable assistance.

On a more personal note, I must thank my husband, Jim, for his love and support, and my parents for instilling in me the belief that any goal can be reached through hard work, a positive attitude, and the determination to succeed.

Preface

When I was a director of nursing in a long-term care facility, the phone call to my office from the receptionist stating that the state surveyors were in the building always caused the same reaction—anxiety! What would they be checking—documentation or resident care? Do I have enough staff on each unit? Are we ready for this inspection? How long will they be here?

I also was concerned about not having a more objective, concrete way of measuring quality care in my nursing center. Just because documentation in the residents' charts was complete or families hadn't been knocking on my office door with complaints for a few weeks, that did not convince me the highest level of quality care was being provided.

In response to similar industry-wide concerns, quality indicators were born. Using information obtained from the Minimum Data Set (MDS), currently 24 specific areas of resident care can be measured and assessed during the survey process. This information is available to long-term care regulators and facility staff—now both groups are able to conduct a preliminary assessment before the state inspection to determine whether quality care is present.

Aside from assisting with the survey process, the quality indicators can also help facilities decide which areas of resident care need to be strengthened.

Quality continues to be an abstract concept; however, the 24 indicators can point nursing homes in the proper direction toward ensuring even better care for our elderly residents.

In 2002 the Centers for Medicare & Medicaid Services (CMS) developed a related use for the MDS data called the quality measures. This data is used to provide quality information to the public so that consumers can make comparisons between nursing homes. These measures are calculated solely from the responses on the MDS form and can be an indication of the presence or absence of quality in a nursing home. The public is now able to view measures of quality for nursing homes in their area before making a choice for nursing home placement. This book discusses the quality measures in Chapter 15.

The book explains the quality indicators, the specific MDS items that affect each indicator, and accurate assessment and coding of these MDS items. Although both the revised *Resident Assessment Instrument User's Manual* and the quality indicator guide from CMS explain the basics of these two areas, I have tried to use this information to develop a concise guide to using the quality indicators not only for good survey results but also to provide even better care.

Because every nursing home staff member should be concerned about providing quality care, all departments in the nursing center will benefit from the information in this book. During my years in long-term care management, not only has the nursing department provided me with much information and many observations but other departments, such a s housekeeping, dietary, and maintenance, also have offered valuable insight into improving quality.

I am pleased to present this second edition of my book. Changes to the *Resident Assessment Instrument User's Manual* that affect the way you code the MDS, plus more knowledge about how quality indicators drive the survey process, gave me the opportunity to draft a newer version of this book. Add the quality measures to the mix, and that adds up to numerous changes between the original and this second edition.

I encourage the reader of this book to use this information as both an overview to quality indicators and as a reference guide to specific areas of concern. I have organized each quality indicator chapter similarly to make it easier to find the specific information required.

Quality of care is a concept not only important in preventing regulatory problems but also vitally necessary in the long-term care environment. Our elderly residents deserve only the best we can offer; we cannot afford to provide any less than the highest quality care possible. We truly have the power to enhance lives and assist in maximizing the potential of each nursing home resident.

Chapter 1

The Quality Indicators: An Overview

What constitutes quality care?

Does your nursing home provide good care? Are you meeting your residents' needs? Are the residents' family members pleased with the service? The answers to questions such as these will help determine whether your nursing home is delivering quality care. Meeting and exceeding quality standards of the Centers for Medicare & Medicaid (CMS) is an ongoing concern for both nursing home staff and long-term care (LTC) regulatory agencies. This book provides tips and practical methods for answering questions about quality care to assist you in providing the best possible care for all of your residents.

How do you define *quality*? Although it has become an important term in the nursing home industry, objectively determining what constitutes quality care in nursing homes can be difficult. Providing quality care means different things for different people; in fact, there are probably as many definitions of quality as there are caretakers. Variables that are often used to measure quality include the following:

- Overall cleanliness and appearance of the building
- Resident and family satisfaction

- Lack of complaints
- Appearance of the residents
- Documentation of care provided
- Adequate and knowledgeable staff members
- Professional medical care treating healthcare needs

To quantitatively measure these and other variables of quality care within nursing homes, LTC regulatory agencies use a variety of methods, including routine and unannounced inspections, complaint investigations (as a response to family and resident concerns), and programs to recognize good nursing homes.

The quality indicators

The quality indicators, developed by CMS in conjunction with the Center for Health Systems Research and Analysis (CHSRA) at the University of Wisconsin-Madison, have become the main tool for assessing whether quality care was provided and the outcome of that care. How do the quality indicators work? How are they different from other forms of assessment? The quality indicators draw on the information from the Minimum Data Set Assessment (MDS). The MDS form allows regulatory agencies to gather consistent, reliable, and valid data from nursing homes across the country. The current MDS (version 2.0) provides a comprehensive assessment of an individual resident's healthcare status, including key information that helps to determine whether the resident received quality care.

The assessment and documentation for the MDS and the resulting quality indicator scores are critical both to the success of your organization and to the delivery of optimum care to your residents. Data from the MDS form is easy to obtain; the forms are transmitted electronically to a designated depository where the information is compiled to monitor specific quality measures.

Scoring the quality indicators: Where does the data come from?
CMS and CHSRA have identified 11 domains, or categories of care, by which to measure quality (Figure 1.1). Each domain contains one or more quality indicators for a total of 24 areas by which CMS objectively measures quality care (Figure 1.2). The information used to score the 24 quality indicators is taken directly from the MDS form. Surveyors sometimes use more than one MDS per resident to determine scores, depending on the indicator type. For example, whereas incidence indicators use the data from two separate MDSs to arrive at a data point, prevalence indicators only take data from one MDS. Incidence indicators include the following:

- New fractures (indicator 1)
- Cognitive impairment (indicator 7)
- Decline in late loss activities of daily living (ADLs) (indicator 17)
- Decline in range of motion (ROM) (indicator 18)

CMS gathers the data for incidence indicators from the most recent MDS and the MDS completed immediately before that assessment. Although these four incidence indicators measure changes in the resident's condition over time, the remaining 20 prevalence indicators measure the resident's current condition, and thus only use data from the most recent MDS assessment.

Figure 1.1

The 11 Quality Domains

1. Accidents
2. Behavioral/emotional patterns
3. Clinical management
4. Cognitive patterns
5. Elimination/incontinence
6. Infection control
7. Nutrition/eating
8. Physical functioning
9. Psychotropic drug use
10. Quality of life
11. Skin care

Figure 1.2

The 24 Quality Indicators

1. Incidence of new fractures
2. Prevalence of falls
3. Prevalence of behavioral symptoms affecting others
4. Prevalence of symptoms of depression
5. Prevalence of symptoms of depression without antidepressant therapy
6. Use of nine or more different medications
7. Incidence of cognitive impairment
8. Prevalence of bladder or bowel incontinence
9. Prevalence of occasional or frequent bladder or bowel incontinence without a toileting plan
10. Prevalence of indwelling catheter
11. Prevalence of fecal impaction
12. Prevalence of urinary tract infections
13. Prevalence of weight loss
14. Prevalence of tube feeding

Figure 1.2 (cont.)

15. Prevalence of dehydration
16. Prevalence of bedfast residents
17. Incidence of decline in late loss ADLs
18. Incidence of decline in ROM
19. Prevalence of antipsychotic use, in the absence of psychotic or related conditions
20. Prevalence of antianxiety/hypnotic use
21. Prevalence of hypnotic use more than two times in last week
22. Prevalence of daily physical restraints
23. Prevalence of little or no activity
24. Prevalence of stage 1–4 pressure ulcers

Risk adjustment

Several of the 24 quality indicators are risk adjusted. For instance, the following prevalence indicators further classify residents into high-risk or low-risk categories:

- Behavioral symptoms affecting others (indicator 3)
- Bladder or bowel incontinence (indicator 8)
- Antipsychotic medication use, in the absence of psychotic or related conditions (indicator 19)
- Stage 1–4 pressure ulcers (indicator 24)

The presence of psychotic disorders, behavior problems, cognitive impairment, dependence in ADLs, or other complex serious medical issues can influence how susceptible a resident is to the development of certain conditions.

Sentinel events

Further definition of the 24 quality indicators includes the identification of three sentinel health events:

- Prevalence of fecal impaction (indicator 11)
- Prevalence of dehydration (indicator 15)
- Prevalence of stage 1–4 pressure ulcers in low-risk residents (indicator 24)

The presence of any one of these conditions in one resident will inevitably prompt a serious investigation.

What causes a quality indicator to flag?

Specific coding from the MDS form determines whether a quality indicator is obtained for each resident. Each quality indicator is directly linked to one or more items on the MDS and will be present depending on the coding of those specific MDS items. A resident will therefore "flag" a quality indicator if the nursing facility codes the MDS according to the numerical definition of the quality indicator.

Where does your facility stand?

To determine the percentage of residents who have flagged a quality indicator, use the following simple formula: Divide the number of residents who have the potential to flag an indicator (the denominator) into the number of residents who have actually flagged that indicator (the numerator). This percentage allows nursing homes to compare themselves to other facilities and receive a percentile ranking. A low percentile rank shows that the nursing home has fewer residents with a particular quality indicator than the average, whereas a nursing home with a high percentile rank would have an above-average number of residents with the quality indicator in question.

Measuring quality

After all of this data is determined, categorized, measured, and interpreted, how do surveyors determine the quality of care? During the LTC survey process, inspectors use this information to identify which areas of care require further investigation. They carefully check quality indicators that have a high percentile rank. Although a high percentile ranking for an indicator does not necessarily indicate a lack of quality, it is a red flag for further investigation. In certain cases, however, the facility's admission policies or care specialization might cause an artificial flag of a quality indicator that should not be considered a sign of poor care.

Educating your clinical team

Because survey success is so closely tied to the MDS assessment process and the quality indicators, it is important for nursing home staff to understand how surveyors obtain and interpret quality indicator information. Scoring well on the quality indicators is crucial to your organization's success. Though most facilities recognize this, there are few references that clearly explain the quality indicators and how they are derived in language that is easy to understand.

How to use this book

This book takes you through all 24 quality indicators and explains the key points, such as the prevalence or incidence of the indicator, the residents used to determine the numerator and denominator, risk adjustment, specific MDS items influencing the indicator, and, finally, accurate coding and assessment of each MDS item. Once you have a thorough understanding of each of the preceding items for each quality indicator, you will be better prepared to deliver and ensure quality care for all of your residents.

Chapter 2

The Minimum Data Set

A care-planning or reimbursement tool?

The Minimum Data Set (MDS) was developed as a standardized tool for the clinical assessment of nursing home residents. The MDS assesses several main areas on a regular scheduled basis, including medical diseases and patient history, nursing care required, psychosocial status, activity involvement, and nutritional needs, so that appropriate planning, implementation, and evaluation of care can be conducted. The MDS was originally created to help facilities gather the necessary clinical information for proper care planning.

However, facilities no longer use the MDS solely for care planning. CMS now uses the information from this form to determine a facility's Medicare payment as well. Under the prospective payment system (PPS), the amount of Medicare Part A reimbursement a nursing facility receives is linked directly to the assessment and coding of care on the MDS form. Today, the financial status of a nursing home depends on accurate and timely completion of these assessments. Not only is the MDS used for clinical and reimbursement purposes, it is also the resident assessment instrument used to obtain the information to measure the 24 quality indicators. In the current financial and regulatory environment, accurate and timely completion of the MDS is crucial to an institution's survival.

Using the MDS effectively

A team-based approach to resident assessment

Ideally, to gain an accurate picture of the resident's healthcare status, facilities should gather input from all of the appropriate departments, including nursing, dietary, social services, activities, and rehabilitation therapy, when completing the MDS form. Facilities also should not underestimate the importance of conducting a face-to-face resident assessment; it is not sufficient to rely solely on documented information in the resident's chart, which provides only part of the picture.

Completing the MDS

When completing the MDS, identify both the time period used for the assessment and the reason for completing the form. The assessment reference date (A3a) or the final day of the look-back period is usually based on a seven-day time frame, unless otherwise indicated. The primary reason for the assessment must be coded in A8a. When a LTC facility admits a new resident, it must complete an initial admission assessment by day 14 of the resident's stay at the nursing home. A quarterly assessment, completed at least every three months, then follows, and the facility completes an annual assessment within 12 months of the initial admission assessment. This cycle of quarterlies and annuals continues for the length of the resident's stay at the nursing home. If nursing home staff find an error on a prior assessment, a correction MDS must be completed. If a resident's condition changes greatly, the facility must complete a significant change in status assessment.

The MDS and the resident assessment protocols

MDSs may be considered full or comprehensive. For a full assessment, facilities only need to complete the MDS form, whereas for a comprehensive assessment, they must submit the MDS form and the resident assessment protocol (RAP) summary (Figure 2.1). The RAP summary is a classification tool used for continued care planning. Specific items on the MDS pertain to each RAP area; the coding of these items determines the extent of this future planning. The admission and annual assessments, a significant change in status, and a significant correction of previous full assessments are all considered comprehensive and require the completion of both the RAP summary and the care plan. However, quarterly assessments and significant corrections of quarterly assessments are not considered comprehensive assessments and therefore do not require RAP summary forms.

The MDS and the quality indicators

After the facility completes the MDS and enters it into a computer program, staff members transmit this information to the appropriate regulatory agency, where it is used to generate quality indicator reports. Six MDS assessments—admission, annual, significant change in status, significant correction of a prior full assessment, quarterly review, and significant correction of a prior quarterly assessment—determine a facility's quality indicator report results. Although the admission assessment does not directly affect quality indicator percentages, it is used for other quality indicator reports.

Figure 2.1

The 18 RAPs

1. Delirium
2. Cognitive loss
3. Visual function
4. Communication
5. ADL functional/rehabilitation potential
6. Urinary incontinence and indwelling catheter
7. Psychosocial well-being
8. Mood state
9. Behavioral symptoms
10. Activities
11. Falls
12. Nutritional status

Figure 2.1 (Cont.)

The 18 RAPs

13. Feeding tube
14. Dehydration/fluid maintenance
15. Dental care
16. Pressure ulcers
17. Psychotropic drug use
18. Physical restraints

Careful coding: Key to success

It is imperative that the MDS accurately reflects the nursing facility's residents and the care provided to those residents. Using proper assessment techniques helps minimize errors on the MDS. Two of the most common errors occur in coding and assessment. Coding errors occur if a staff member misreads the form and enters an improper value in a specific section, or if someone keys a value incorrectly when the information is transcribed into the computer program. Nursing facilities should not rely exclusively on their computer program's auditing feature. Instead, nursing home staff members should ensure not only that all values entered on the MDS are within the appropriate code range of values allowed by each item, but also that staff members correctly enter this data into the computer. Staff members should check hard copies of the MDS and verify information to ensure accuracy.

Avoiding assessment errors

Assessment errors are more difficult to define and determine than coding errors and often occur when the assessor either does not understand what information the MDS requests or does not know how to assess for the information. First, understand exactly what specific information the MDS requests. Reread the items and answering instructions several times, paying close attention to key words. Refer to the revised *Resident Assessment Instrument User's Manual* to determine how to code a response. Nurses who are new to the job and unfamiliar with the MDS should consider attending MDS training seminars. The MDS is lengthy and complex, especially for staff members inexperienced with its completion.

CMS derives quality indicator data solely from the MDS; therefore, nursing home staff must understand the importance of the accuracy of this assessment. If staff members do not complete the MDS properly, quality indicator scores may indicate to regulatory surveyors the presence of a care problem that does not exist. If incorrect quality indicators result in survey discrepancies, inspectors may penalize the facility because of inaccurate assessment of residents. When checking both the quality indicators and the accuracy of the MDS, surveyors may identify other areas needing special attention and write deficiencies based on incorrect assessments.

Helpful tools

The chapters that follow discuss each of the quality indicators and include information on how to accurately assess and code the MDS items that pertain to each indicator. At the conclusion of each domain chapter, a table provides an at-a-glance summary of the MDS items and the specific MDS coding affecting each quality indicator. Use these tables as quick reference guides for the material covered in each of the chapters.

Additionally, Figure 2.2 lists all sections and items of the MDS form that pertain to the quality indicators, as well as the number of the specific indicator affected by each MDS item. This list is a cross-reference to the information presented in the tables following each chapter.

As you read through this book and refer to the accompanying tables and figures, you will come to understand the critical importance of accurate assessment of nursing home residents. Coding just one MDS item incorrectly can negatively affect the scoring for several quality indicators. Completion of the MDS form is no longer purely paper compliance; the MDS drives the success or failure of LTC facilities in today's regulatory environment.

Figure 2.2

MDS Items and Affected Quality Indicators

MDS Item	Quality Indicator(s) Affected*
Section B	
B1: Comatose	4, 5, 8, 17, 23, and 24
B2a: Short-term memory	3, 7, 8, and 19
B4: Cognitive skills for daily decision making	3, 7, 8, and 19
Section E	
E1a: Resident made negative statements	4 and 5
E1g: Recurrent statements that something terrible is about to happen	4 and 5
E1j: Unpleasant mood in the morning	4 and 5
E1n: Repetitive physical movements	4 and 5
E1o: Withdrawal from activities of interest	4 and 5
E1p: Reduced social interaction	4 and 5
E2: Mood persistence	4 and 5
E4b Box A: Verbally abusive behavioral symptoms frequency	3 and 19
E4c Box A: Physically abusive behavioral symptoms frequency	3 and 19
E4d Box A: Socially inappropriate/disruptive behavioral symptoms frequency	3 and 19
E4e Box A: Resists care frequency	4 and 5

Figure 2.2 (Cont.)

MDS Items and Affected Quality Indicators

Section G

G1a Box A: Bed mobility self-performance ....8, 17, and 24
G1b Box A: Transfer self-performance ....8, 17, and 24
G1c Box A: Walk in room self-performance 17
G1d Box A: Walk in corridor self-performance 17
G1e Box A: Locomotion on unit self-performance ....8 and 17
G1f Box A: Locomotion off unit self-performance 17
G1g Box A: Dressing self-performance 17
G1h Box A: Eating self-performance 17
G1i Box A: Toilet use self-performance 17
G1j Box A: Personal hygiene self-performance 17
G4a Box A: Neck ROM 18
G4b Box A: Arm ROM 18
G4c Box A: Hand ROM 18
G4d Box A: Leg ROM 18
G4e Box A: Foot ROM 18
G4f Box A: Other ROM 18
G6a: Bedfast all or most of the time 16

Section H

H1a: Bowel continence ....8 and 9
H1b: Bladder continence ....8 and 9
H2d: Fecal impaction 11

Figure 2.2 (Cont.)

MDS Items and Affected Quality Indicators

H3a: Any scheduled toileting plan 9
H3b: Bladder retraining program .9
H3d: Indwelling catheter . . . . .8 and 10
H3i: Ostomy present 8

Section I

I1ff: Manic depression 3
I1gg: Schizophrenia . . . . .3, 19, and 20
I2j: Urinary tract infection in last 30 days 12
I3: Other current or more detailed diagnoses . . . . .3, 15, 19, 20, and 24
and International Classification of Diseases,
Ninth Revision (ICD-9) codes

Section J

J1c: Dehydrated; output exceeds input 15
J1i: Hallucinations . . . . .19 and 20
J4a: Fell in past 30 days 2
J4c: Hip fracture in the last 180 days 1
J4d: Other fracture in the last 180 days 1
J5c: End-stage disease, six or fewer months 24
to live

Section K

K3a: Weight change—weight loss . . . . .4, 5, and 13
K5b: Feeding tube 14

Figure 2.2 (Cont.)

MDS Items and Affected Quality Indicators

Section M

M2a: Pressure ulcer 24

Section N

N1a: Awake in the morning . . . . .4 and 5

N1b: Awake in the afternoon . . . . .4 and 5

N1c: Awake in the evening . . . . .4 and 5

N1d: No time awake . . . . .4 and 5

N2: Average time involved in activities 23

Section O

O1: Number of medications 6

O4a: Antipsychotic 19

O4b: Antianxiety 20

O4c: Antidepressant 5

O4d: Hypnotic . . . . .20 and 21

Section P

P4c: Trunk restraint 22

P4d: Limb restraint 22

P4e: Chair prevents rising 22

*See Figure 1.2 on p. 5 for a complete list of the quality indicators that correspond to the numbers in column 2.

Chapter 3

Accidents Domain

The first domain identified by CMS—accidents—includes two quality indicators: incidence of new fractures and prevalence of falls. The majority of nursing home residents are elderly and are more susceptible to falls and fractures because of their advanced age and compromising medical conditions. Because of this, regulatory agencies carefully monitor the measures taken to prevent falls as well as the number of accidents in long-term care (LTC) facilities. Falls and fractures are often incapacitating and can exacerbate existing medical difficulties; therefore, accident prevention is crucial to maintaining the resident's independence and health status. Associated concerns in this domain include the presence of environmental safety hazards, over-medication of residents, too few staff members, and inappropriate restraint use.

Quality indicator 1: Incidence of new fractures

Basic information

- **Indicator type:** New fractures is an incidence indicator, meaning that the change in a resident's condition is measured over time. This indicator considers the data from the current MDS (excluding the initial admission assessment) and the previous MDS to determine whether a new fracture has occurred.

- **Facility percentage:** Surveyors analyze the facility percentage, which is calculated by comparing all residents identified on the current assessment as having a new fracture to residents identified on the previous assessment as not having a fracture.

- **Risk adjustment:** Quality indicator 1 is not risk adjusted.

Related MDS items

The two MDS items relating to fractures are hip fracture in last 180 days (J4c) and other fracture in last 180 days (J4d). Either of the following scenarios will cause this quality indicator to be present:

- J4c is checked on the current MDS assessment and not checked on the prior MDS assessment.

- J4d is checked on the current MDS assessment and not checked on the prior MDS assessment.

Because the type of fracture is not specified in the title of this quality indicator, either a new hip fracture or a new fracture of any other bone will cause this indicator to flag. Only one of the preceding scenarios needs to be present to result in recognition of the quality indicator.

MDS assessment and coding

Although most MDS items apply to the resident's status during the previous seven days, items J4c and J4d are exceptions. Both of these items require caregivers to identify hip fractures or other fractures that have occurred within the past 180 days. It is important to count actual days rather than to consider just the previous six-month period. For instance, a fracture that occurred exactly six months ago might not necessarily fall within the 180-day period and therefore should not be checked on the MDS. Additionally, if a resident is a new admission or has not been in the nursing facility for 180 days, then the assessor must review for fractures the entire previous 180 days, including the time before admission. In this case, it is necessary to obtain adequate medical information from previous health facilities or through conversations with the resident, family members, or other people familiar with the resident.

Documentation for fractures should include the exact date on which the fracture occurred, not just the month and year, so that staff members can accurately assess and code. After reviewing all pertinent information, staff should check the appropriate box—or boxes—if fractures did occur. If a facility has a high percentage of new fractures, further investigation is warranted to determine the cause and whether prevention is possible.

Quality indicator 2: Prevalence of falls

Basic information

- **Indicator type:** Unlike quality indicator 1, quality indicator 2 is classified as a prevalence indicator, so surveyors use the information generated from only the current MDS assessment (excluding the initial admission assessment).

- **Facility percentage:** Surveyors analyze the nursing home percentage, which is calculated by comparing the number of residents coded as having fallen with all other residents who have a completed MDS assessment in the nursing facility.

- **Risk adjustment:** Quality indicator 2 is not risk adjusted.

Related MDS item

Only one item on the MDS specifically relates to falls and to this indicator: fell in last 30 days (J4a). If this item is checked on the current MDS assessment, the quality indicator will flag.

MDS assessment and coding

Fell in last 30 days (J4a) is another exception to the seven-day assessment rule. It is important to count the actual number of days rather than considering just one month before the assessment reference date of the MDS. A month before the assessment might be 31 days, and the fall would not be included. If a resident was admitted less than 30 days ago, the entire 30-day time period must be considered; therefore, it is necessary to review any admitting documentation that came with the resident and any verbal information provided by the resident and family members, or both. Also note that if item J4b—fell in last 31–180 days—is applicable, it will not influence the flagging of this quality indicator. Only recent falls are included.

Additionally, a fracture within the designated time period does not automatically mean that the resident has fallen; fractures in the elderly can occur in the absence of a fall. If a resident did fall within the designated 30-day time frame, however, check the box at item J4a. A high number of falls will cause surveyors to explore whether these falls were preventable or if safety hazards, such as clutter in hallways and in resident rooms, compromised the quality of care provided.

At a Glance

Domain #1
Accidents

Quality Indicators	MDS Items	MDS Codes
1. Incidence of new fractures	J4c: Hip fracture in last 180 days	Box is checked on current MDS and not checked on previous MDS, or;
	J4d: Other fracture in last 180 days	Box is checked on current MDS and not checked on previous MDS
2. Prevalence of falls	J4a: Fell in past 30 days	Box is checked

Chapter 4

Behavioral/Emotional Patterns Domain

The behavioral and emotional patterns domain is of great concern for many nursing homes, because diminished mental capacity and psychological conditions such as depression can be common in their elderly residents. Organic brain syndrome, senile dementia, and Alzheimer's disease are just a few of the major illnesses that afflict the geriatric population and directly influence a resident's behavioral status. Three quality indicators are included under this domain:

- Prevalence of behavioral symptoms affecting others
- Prevalence of symptoms of depression
- Prevalence of symptoms of depression without antidepressant medication

These three quality indicators measure the extent of behavioral and emotional problems and the presence or absence of quality intervention and evaluation of care.

Quality indicator 3: Prevalence of behavioral symptoms affecting others

Basic information

- **Indicator type:** Because quality indicator 3 is a prevalence indicator, surveyors use the data generated from the current MDS assessment (excluding the initial admission assessment).
- **Facility percentage:** Surveyors analyze the facility percentage, which is calculated by identifying the number of residents coded as having behavioral symptoms affecting others compared with all other residents with a completed MDS assessment in the nursing facility.
- **Risk adjustment:** Quality indicator 3 is the first of the 24 indicators to be risk adjusted. CMS classifies all residents who have behavioral symptoms affecting others in either a high-risk or low-risk category. The risk factor section of this chapter discusses the determination of this classification.

Related MDS items

Verbally abusive behavior (E4b), physically abusive behavior (E4c), and socially inappropriate or disruptive behavior (E4d) provide the information for this indicator. However, only column A—the behavioral symptom frequency—directly affects the quality indicator. Alterability of behavioral symptoms coding in column B has no bearing on indicator data. Therefore, if any one of the following three scenarios is present, the resident will flag for behavioral symptoms affecting others:

- E4b box A is coded as a 1, 2, or 3
- E4c box A is coded as a 1, 2, or 3
- E4d box A is coded as a 1, 2, or 3

Assessors determine the codes for these items by the frequency of the behavior. If the specific behavior did not occur at all within the seven-day assessment period, they code the item as a 0; if the behavior occurred 1–3 days in the seven-day assessment period, they code the behavior as a 1; if the behavior occurred on 4–6 days, they code the item as a 2; and if the behavior occurred all seven days, they code the behavior as a 3.

Weighing the risk factor

The risk adjustment for quality indicator 3 causes surveyors to consider more MDS items, which relate to the identification of a potential problem with behavioral symptoms.

High-risk residents

Cognitive impairment

CHSRA has defined the presence of cognitive impairment as the first of two areas that can classify a resident as high risk. Two MDS items—cognitive skills for daily decision making (B4) and short-term memory (B2a)—can place a resident in either a high-risk or low-risk category for behavioral symptoms. You must code both of these items as follows for cognitive impairment to be present:

- B4 is coded as a 1, 2, or 3
- B2a is coded as a 1

As explained on the MDS form, code item B4 as a 0 if the resident makes proper and reasonable decisions independently; use a code of 1 for modified independence; code 2 designates moderate impairment; and code 3 indicates severe impairment. Item B2a pertains to a resident's short-term memory; code a 0 if the resident's memory appears good, or code it as a 1 if the resident has a memory problem.

Psychotic disorders

The second area defined by CHSRA that could place a resident in the high-risk category is the presence of psychotic disorders such as schizophrenia or manic depression. Code these conditions in section I, disease diagnoses, of the MDS. Specifically, if you check manic depression (I1ff) or schizophrenia (I1gg), the resident is placed in the high-risk category.

Additionally, information from other current or more detailed diagnoses (I3) can categorize the patient as high-risk. According to CHSRA, any diagnosis with an ICD-9 CM (International Classification of Diseases, 9th revision, Clinical Modification) code of 295.00 through 295.9, 297.00 through 298.9, or 296.00 through 296.9 results in this high-risk classification. Examples of diagnoses within these groupings include paranoid states, delusional disorders, depressive psychoses, bipolar affective disorders, and affective psychoses.

Usually, CMS uses the most recent MDS assessment to obtain this diagnosis information; however, an exception occurs with this risk adjustment. Items I1ff and I1gg are not included as part of the quarterly assessment; therefore, if the most recent assessment is a quarterly assessment, the most recent full or complete MDS is used.

Low-risk residents

If the resident does not have any of the indicators of high risk (for example, cognitive impairment, psychotic disorders, or manic depression), the resident is in the low-risk category.

MDS assessment and coding

Many MDS items pertain to quality indicator 3. You must accurately assess and code all of these items to reflect the behavioral status of the resident.

Behavioral symptoms

Section E4, behavioral symptoms, assesses the resident's behaviors during a seven-day period. Resident behaviors may be more prevalent during certain periods; however, staff members should consider only the previous seven days for this assessment. Nurses' notes, social service progress notes, and activity progress notes can all include valuable documentation of behavioral symptoms to complete this assessment. Consultations with mental health professionals can also yield pertinent information about behaviors.

Direct observation of the residents' behaviors is the most accurate method of properly assessing this area. The nurse completing the MDS should consult with staff from all shifts who observe the residents' behaviors, because often, residents with impaired mental functioning exhibit more inappropriate behaviors during the evening than during the day. Thus, if you do not review the documented observations from all shifts before coding the MDS, the MDS form may not reflect the resident's behavioral status.

Inappropriate behaviors

Verbally abusive behaviors (E4b) can include yelling loudly at staff and other residents, using foul language, and inappropriate calling out. Physically abusive behaviors (E4c) include striking out at other residents and staff members, kicking, and sexual abuse. Socially inappropriate/disruptive behaviors (E4d) are those actions considered unacceptable in comparison to social norms and standards, including public displays of sexual behavior, throwing items at staff and residents, going through other residents' belongings, and abusive gestures toward staff and other residents.

The risk adjustment for quality indicator 3 causes both surveyors and the nursing facility to consider additional MDS items affecting the indicator outcome. As discussed above, cognitive impairment is assessed by the ability or inability to make decisions and the presence or absence of memory problems. Assess both of these areas by reviewing chart documentation, observing and interacting with the resident, and questioning other staff members, including non-nursing personnel. Social workers and activity staff who interact with the resident in nonmedical social situations can provide valuable insight into the resident's cognitive abilities. Involved family members also can provide information to help properly code these areas.

Cognitive skills for daily decision making

Cognitive skills for daily decision making (B4) addresses residents' ability to make decisions in their current environment. Do not assess a resident's ability to make major life-changing decisions outside of the nursing home environment; instead, carefully monitor everyday decisions regarding, for example, what clothes to wear or which activities to attend. Accurate coding of this item in the range from independent to severely impaired depends on assessing how a resident deals with his or her daily routine and the amount of staff intervention the resident needs to perform routine tasks. Nursing assistants, because of the extent of their patient contact and the direct hands-on care they give residents, have the most information about a resident's daily routine, so they are generally the caretakers most qualified to make accurate assessments.

Short-term memory

Short-term memory (B2a) assesses the resident's ability to remember events that have occurred in the recent past. The assessor can use structured memory tests to question the resident about recent happenings or activities. If a resident is unable to recall certain information, the assessor should code the resident as having a memory problem. Family members are usually aware of the resident's memory changes over time, so caretakers should use them as a resource when trying to determine whether a resident has a memory problem.

Disease diagnoses

Specific disease diagnoses also influence the risk adjustment for quality indicator 3. Manic depression and schizophrenia are already listed in section I, disease diagnoses, and you should check them if either of these conditions are active diagnoses and relate to the resident's current health status. Diagnoses that were present years ago but do not currently affect any area of the resident's health status do not need to be checked in section I1 or written in I3. Geriatric residents often have an extensive list of diagnoses, but all of these may not be applicable to their current status.

Obtain diagnostic information at the time of admission from the hospital transfer paperwork or from a completed history and physical form. As new conditions develop, update this diagnoses list. As discussed above, psychotic disorders such as schizophrenic disorders, paranoid states, and other affective psychoses influence the risk adjustment and should be written in I3 if present.

If many residents who are at low risk for inappropriate behavioral symptoms exhibit these conditions, the facility should determine whether their behavior was preventable. In certain cases, the facility's admitting practices might influence which types of residents it accepts. If a facility admits a large number of residents with a documented history of inappropriate behavior, they can expect to have more behavioral issues. Facilities should examine trends in inappropriate behavior to determine why they occur.

Quality indicator 4: Prevalence of symptoms of depression

Basic information

- **Indicator type:** The second indicator in the behavioral and emotional patterns domain, quality indicator 4, is also a prevalence indicator. Surveyors use information generated from the current MDS (excluding the initial admission assessment) to determine the facility's percentage.

- **Facility percentage:** Surveyors analyze the facility percentage, which is calculated by identifying the number of residents with symptoms of depression compared with all other residents in the facility that have a completed MDS assessment.
- **Risk adjustment:** Quality indicator 4 is not risk adjusted.

Related MDS items

MDS section E provides most of the data for this quality indicator. Mood persistence (E2), coded as either a 1 or 2, is the first MDS item that affects this indicator. The MDS form states that if one or more of the 16 mood indicators of depression, anxiety, or sadness (E1) is present, you should code item E2 as a 1 if the depression or sadness was easily altered or a 2 if the mood indicators were not easily altered. This item looks at the persistence of mood indicators over a seven-day period. If the resident was depressed because of an event that occurred some time ago but has not displayed any mood indicators within the previous seven days, the code for this item is 0.

The second aspect in determining whether a resident has depression is the presence of two or more of the five symptoms of depression identified by CHSRA (Figure 4.1).

MDS assessment and coding

Quality indicator 4 is more complex and confusing than others because of the number of MDS items that cause the indicator to flag. To review, a persistent sad mood in addition to at least two of the five symptoms of depression in Figure 4.1 causes the indicator to flag.

Mood persistence

Assess mood persistence (E2) by observing whether the resident exhibited a sad or depressed mood during the previous seven days. Do not assess a persistent elated or happy mood on its own, even if evident over the assessment period. However, if the resident exhibits an elated mood in combination with depression, as is the case with bipolar disorders such as manic depression, you should code the mood in E2. Direct interaction with the resident; visual cues of depression, such as a sad facial expression or crying; and discussions with staff members and family can help caretakers determine whether the resident exhibits a depressed mood. The presence of any of the 16 items in E1 is an indication of sadness and a depressed mood. It is then necessary to determine whether this staff interaction and reassurance could or could not alter this mood. A resident might exhibit several of the indicators listed in E1; however, after the resident talks with staff or family, these sad emotions might diminish. Conversely, a resident could remain depressed even after repeated attempts at reassurance.

When coding E2, use only a seven-day assessment period. When coding E1, however, assess the previous 30-day period. Therefore, indicators that are present in E1 might not affect the coding of E2 if these indicators occurred before the seven-day assessment period. Six of the 16 items in E1 can affect this quality indicator of depression: E1a, E1g, E1j, E1n, E1o, and E1p. These items relate to the five symptoms of depression (see Figure 4.1) and should be coded according to frequency of occurrence. If a resident exhibits an item in E1 only one time during the 30-day assessment period up to five times per week, the code would be a 1; you should code six to seven times per week a 2. Once again, to assess this item accurately, it is critical to obtain information from staff and family members who are in frequent contact with the resident and who are able to accurately relate information about the resident's mood.

Figure 4.1

Symptoms of Depression

If at least two of the following five symptoms of depression are present, combined with the sad mood identified in E2, surveyors will flag this indicator. The five symptoms and the associated MDS items include the following:

1. **Distress:** E1a (resident made negative statements) coded as a 1 (exhibited up to 5 days a week) or 2 (exhibited 6–7 days a week).

2. **Agitation or withdrawal:** E1n (repetitive physical movements) coded as a 1 (exhibited up to 5 days a week) or 2 (exhibited 6–7 days a week); or E4e box A (behavioral symptom of resisting care) coded as a 1 (behavior occurred 1–3 days in the previous 7 days), a 2 (behavior occurred 4–6 days of the previous 7 days), or a 3 (behavior occurred daily in the previous 7 days); or E1o (withdrawal from activities of interest) coded as a 1 (exhibited up to 5 days a week) or a 2 (exhibited 6–7 days a week); or E1p (reduced social interaction) coded as a 1 (exhibited up to 5 days a week) or a 2 (exhibited 6–7 days a week).

3. **Wake with unpleasant mood:** E1j (unpleasant mood in the morning) coded as a 1 (exhibited up to 5 days a week) or 2 (exhibited 6–7 days a week); or N1d (resident is not awake during the day) is checked or the resident is awake only during the morning, afternoon, or evening and is not comatose, in which case, only one or no check marks are made for awake periods N1a (awake during the morning), N1b (awake during the afternoon), or N1c (awake during the evening); and B1 (comatose) coded as 0.

Figure 4.1 (cont.)

4. Suicidal or recurrent thoughts of death: E1g (recurrent statements that something terrible is about to happen) coded as a 1 (exhibited up to 5 days a week) or a 2 (exhibited 6–7 days a week).

5. Weight loss: K3a (a weight loss of 5% or more in the last 30 days, or 10% or more in the last 180 days) coded as a 1.

Resisting of care

Resisting of care (E4e box A) can also indicate depression. A resident's refusal of food, fluids, medications, or needed assistance from staff members should alert the caretaker that the resident may be depressed. Caretakers should observe these behaviors during the past seven-day period; they can assess the frequency of these behaviors by noting any documentation of refusals and by questioning both the resident and staff.

Time awake

The amount of time a resident spends awake is an excellent indication of depression. Depressed residents might suddenly sleep all of the time or, conversely, be unable to sleep because of intense sadness. Time awake (N1) assesses three time periods in the day during which the resident was not sleeping for more than one hour in the course of the previous seven-day period. Morning is defined as the time the resident awakens until noon; afternoon is noon until 5 p.m.; and evening is 5 p.m. until the resident's bedtime. If a resident is not awake during any of these periods or is awake during only one period (and is not comatose), he or she may be depressed. It can be difficult to determine whether a comatose resident is either awake or alert; therefore, being comatose combined with not being awake is not considered an accurate symptom of depression.

Weight loss

The final symptom of depression and the last MDS item that affects this indicator is weight loss (K3a). You should score this item as a 1 if the resident has lost 5% or more of his or her total weight in the last 30 days or 10% or more of his or her total weight in the last 180 days. Again, it is important to count actual days rather than a one-month or six-month period, because weight losses exactly one or six months ago might not fall within the 30-day and 180-day time frames.

A resident's decreased appetite or refusal of food may indicate that he or she is depressed. Loss of weight and a poor appetite can also play a role in various other conditions, including electrolyte imbalance, cardiac irregularities, and the development of malnutrition. If a resident has the specified percentages of weight loss, you should code item K3a as a 1.

A high percentage of residents with symptoms of depression could indicate either that the facility is not providing appropriate treatment or that the facility specializes in the care of residents with mood disorders and thus has a higher percentage of depressed residents. Determine the reason for the high percentage of depressed residents to help define whether quality of care is present.

Quality indicator 5: Prevalence of symptoms of depression without antidepressant therapy

Basic information

- **Indicator type:** Quality indicator 5 is identical to the previous indicator with one addition: the presence or absence of antidepressant therapy. The indicator is a prevalence indicator using information obtained from the most recently completed MDS assessment (excluding the initial admission assessment).

- **Facility percentage:** Surveyors analyze the facility percentage by comparing those residents with symptoms of depression and no documented antidepressant therapy with all residents in the facility who have a completed MDS assessment.

- **Risk adjustment:** Quality indicator 5 is not risk adjusted.

Related MDS items

The symptoms of depression (E1), mood persistence (E2), resisting of care (E4e), periods of being awake (N1), and weight loss (K3a) all affect quality indicator 5 in the same way that they did for the previous indicator (prevalence of symptoms of depression). One addition should be considered: If the coded responses on a resident's MDS trigger quality indicator 4, the resident will also flag for quality indicator 5 if the facility is not providing antidepressant therapy. Antidepressant (O4c) coded as a 0 indicates the facility did not administer antidepressants during the seven-day assessment period.

MDS assessment and coding

As mentioned on p.42, all coding and assessment guidelines for quality indicator 4 also apply to quality indicator 5. However, for quality indicator 5, you should also code item O4c for administration of antidepressant medication and score it depending on the number of days during the previous seven-day period that the resident actually received antidepressants. Therefore, the range of values for this item is 0 to 7. Assess only the number of days the resident received an antidepressant, not the number of doses. For example, if a resident received a twice daily (b.i.d.) dose of an antidepressant three times weekly, the score would be a 3, not a 6. Given the amount of psychoactive medications available, antidepressants must be distinguished from antianxiety, antipsychotic, and hypnotic medication. A reference book such as the *Physicians' Desk Reference* (*PDR*) or consultation with a pharmacist can assist in classifying the psychoactive medication correctly.

Per the MDS guidelines, antidepressants should be coded as received even if during the seven-day period, the place of administration of the drug is not the nursing facility. If a resident was in a hospital emergency room and documentation indicates the administration of an antidepressant, that dose should be counted in the number of days for the final total in item O4c. If a resident is a new admission, and part of the assessment period is before the nursing home admission, include any antidepressants administered before the admission if there is supporting documentation.

If a resident is coded as a 0 in item O4c and has the symptoms of depression identified in the quality indicator 4 discussion, the resident will also flag for this quality indicator. This does not necessarily mean that quality of care is not present; a resident could be experiencing a brief, situational depression and might not require an antidepressant. If a facility is not administering antidepressant therapy to residents with symptoms of depression, further exploration is needed to determine whether treatment should be provided. Because depression can be common among the elderly, accurate identification and evaluation is important for ensuring an improved quality of life.

At a Glance

Domain #2
Behavioral/Emotional Patterns

Quality Indicators	MDS Items	MDS Codes
3. Prevalence of behavioral symptoms affecting others	E4b Box A: Verbally abusive behavioral symptoms frequency	1, 2, or 3, or;
	E4c Box A: Physically abusive behavioral symptoms frequency	1, 2, or 3, or;
	E4d Box A: Socially inappropriate/disruptive behavioral symptoms frequency	1, 2, or 3
High risk for QI #3	B4: Cognitive skills for daily decision-making	1, 2, or 3, and;
	B2a: Short-term memory	1
	OR	
	I1ff: Manic depression	Box is checked, or;

Domain #2 (cont.)

Quality Indicators	MDS Items	MDS Codes
See previous page.	Igg: Schizophrenia	Box is checked, or;
	I3: Other current or more detailed diagnoses and ICD-9 codes	Diagnosis ICD-9 code is 295.00-295.9, 296.00-296.9, or 297.00-298.9
Low risk for QI #3—All other residents not classified as high risk	N/A	N/A
4. Prevalence of symptoms of depression	E2: Mood persistence	1 or 2 (and at least 2 of the 5 symptoms of depression listed in column 2)
	Symptom 1: E1a: Resident made negative statements	1 or 2
	Symptom 2: E1n: Repetitive physical movements	1 or 2, or;
	E4e Box A: Resists care frequency	1, 2, or 3, or;

Domain #2 (cont.)

Quality Indicators	MDS Items	MDS Codes
See previous page.	E1o: Withdrawal from activities of interest	1 or 2, or;
	E1p: Reduced social interaction	1 or 2
	Symptom 3:	
	E1j: Unpleasant mood in the morning	1 or 2, or;
	N1d: No time awake	Box is checked, or;
	N1a: Awake in the morning; N1b: Awake in the afternoon; N1c: Awake in the evening	Only one or none of the three boxes is checked
	B1: Comatose	0 (in combination with only one or none of N1a, N1b, or N1c checked)
	Symptom 4:	
	E1g: Recurrent statements that something terrible is about to happen	1 or 2

Domain #2 (cont.)

Quality Indicators	MDS Items	MDS Codes
See previous page.	**Symptom 5:**	
	K3a: weight change-weight loss	1
5. Prevalence of symptoms of depression without antidepressant therapy	O4c: Antidepressant	0
	AND	
	E2: Mood persistence	1 or 2 (and at least 2 of the 5 symptoms of depression listed in column 2)
	Symptom 1:	
	E1a: Resident made negative statements	1 or 2
	Symptom 2:	
	E1n: Repetitive physical movements	1 or 2, or;
	E4e Box A: Resists care frequency	1, 2, or 3, or;

Domain #2 (cont.)

Quality Indicators	MDS Items	MDS Codes
See previous page.	E1o: Withdrawal from activities of interest	1 or 2, or;
	E1p: Reduced social interaction	1 or 2
	Symptom 3:	
	E1j: Unpleasant mood in morning	1 or 2, or;
	N1d: No time awake	Box is checked, or;
	N1a: Awake in the morning; N1b: Awake in the afternoon; N1c: Awake in the evening	Only one or none of the three boxes is checked
	B1: Comatose	0 (in combination with only one or none of N1a, N1b, or N1c checked)
	Symptom 4:	
	E1g: Recurrent statements that something terrible is about to happen	1 or 2

Domain #2 (cont.)

Quality Indicators	MDS Items	MDS Codes
See previous page.	**Symptom 5:** K3a: Weight change-weight loss	1

Chapter 5

Clinical Management Domain

Proper management of clinical conditions is vital for quality of care. The elderly in nursing homes frequently have complex needs and more than one disease, but the benefits of extensive treatment must be weighed against the risks of adverse drug interactions. The clinical management domain includes only one quality indicator that pertains to the use of medications. Although other methods could be used to assess clinical management of diseases, such as frequency of physician visits, content of physician's and nurse's progress notes, and history and physical documentation, the use or overuse of medications is one of the more objective methods for determining the appropriate management of diseases.

Quality indicator 6: Use of nine or more different medications

Basic information

- **Indicator type:** Although the title of quality indicator 6 is the only one that does not mention incidence or prevalence, the indicator does consider information from only the most recent MDS completed (excluding the initial admission assessment) to determine the indicator facility outcome.

- **Facility percentage:** Surveyors analyze the facility percentage, which is calculated by comparing residents who received at least nine different medications as recorded on the MDS compared with all residents in the facility who have completed MDS assessments.

- **Risk adjustment:** Quality indicator 6 is not risk adjusted.

Related MDS item

Information from only one MDS item is associated with quality indicator 6: O1, number of medications. Assessors record the number of different medications administered during the seven-day assessment period for this item. The allowable range of values is from 0 (no medication administered) to whatever number of medications was given; there is no upper limit for coding this item.

MDS assessment and coding

Number of medications administered

When determining the number of medications administered, the key concept to consider is the coding of different medications. If a resident received two different doses of the same medication, only count one medication. For example, a resident receiving a specific number of units of insulin in the morning and a different number of units of the same insulin in the afternoon would only be receiving one medication.

Medications received by any route of administration can be counted. Oral, sublingual, intramuscular, intravenous, subcutaneous, rectal, topical, inhalation, and via enteral tube are all accepted routes for this item's coding. Medications also do not have to be obtained only by prescription; also consider over-the-counter medications, such as vitamins and ointments, when determining the total number. Any medications given on an "as needed" or prn basis qualify, as do one-time-only stat doses.

It is best to obtain information about the number of medications administered by referring to the resident's medication and treatment administration records, rather than the physician order sheets. Using the assessment reference date as the final day in the seven-day look-back period, count the number of different medications administered and record this number in box O1. If a resident has a physician order for a medication but it is not given (for example, because of resident refusal or inappropriate vital sign parameters), do not count this medication in the final total.

Polypharmacy

Polypharmacy, or excessive use of many different medications, continues to concern the long-term care industry. Because the elderly resident can have a slower metabolism and therefore medications remain in the body for an extended period, administration of many drugs can quickly cause a build-up of these agents. As the number of medications increases, the risk of adverse side effects also grows. It is well-documented that discontinuing medications may in fact result in greater effectiveness in clinical management of diseases.

A facility with a high proportion of residents receiving nine or more medications does not necessarily mean it does not have quality clinical management. It may indeed indicate an excessive use of medications, or the facility might have many residents with complex disease patterns. Further investigation should determine the reason for the high number of medications administered.

At a Glance

Domain #3
Clinical Management

Quality Indicators	MDS Items	MDS Codes
6. Use of nine or more different medications	O1: Number of medications	9 or higher

Chapter 6

Cognitive Patterns Domain

The ability to perceive surroundings and use reasoning and intuition significantly affects quality of life and influences physical condition. As discussed in Chapter 4, senile dementia and Alzheimer's disease are major concerns in nursing homes. Long-term care facilities must diagnose these problems and provide appropriate evaluation and intervention to maintain the highest possible functional level in residents. One quality indicator is addressed in this domain: incidence of cognitive impairment. Monitoring the development of cognitive difficulties over time can reveal quality-of-care issues and assist in devising appropriate treatment plans.

Quality indicator 7: Incidence of cognitive impairment

Basic information

- **Indicator type:** Quality indicator 7 is the second of four incidence indicators that address a change in resident condition over time. Incidence indicators compare two MDS assessments and note any changes in the coding of specific items. This indicator considers both the current MDS assessment (excluding the initial admission assessment) and the prior MDS assessment to identify whether cognitive impairment has developed.

- **Facility percentage:** Surveyors analyze the facility percentage, which is calculated by identifying those residents on the current MDS coded as having cognitive impairment and comparing them to residents on the prior MDS assessment who did not have cognitive impairment. Residents coded as cognitively impaired on both the current MDS and the prior MDS are not included for the determination of this percentage.

- **Risk adjustment:** Quality indicator 7 is not risk adjusted.

Related MDS items

CHSRA defines cognitive impairment as decision-making impairment and short-term memory difficulty. This definition of cognitive impairment was used previously in the risk adjustment for quality indicator 3 (prevalence of behavioral symptoms affecting others). To review, two MDS items influence the flagging of this cognitive impairment indicator. Staff must code both cognitive skills for daily decision making (B4) and short-term memory (B2a) as follows for this indicator to flag:

- B4 is coded as a 1, 2, or 3

- B2a is coded as a 1

The MDS form specifies the following coding for B4:

- 0 for independent decision making

- 1 for modified independence

- 2 for moderate impairment
- 3 for a resident with severely impaired decision-making abilities

Code item B2a as a 0 if the resident appears to have a good short-term memory or a 1 if the resident has memory problems. Coding of both items B4 and B2a reflects the seven-day period up to and including the assessment reference date.

MDS assessment and coding

Despite the temptation to assess the overall, long-term cognitive status of a resident, it is important to assess only what has occurred during the previous seven-day period, rather than scoring the items according to the staff's perceptions of a resident's gradual decline or improvement over time.

Daily decision making

When determining the code for cognitive skills for daily decision making (B4), use documentation of any difficulties during the assessment period as well as direct observation of the resident and consultation with staff and family members. The nursing home resident could also provide valuable insight about his or her decision-making abilities. As discussed previously (see Chapter 4, Quality Indicator 3), assess only everyday decisions made in the current environment. The numerical score for this item ranges from complete independence to total dependence on staff for decision making. It is important to determine to what degree, if any, the impairment is present so that you code this item accurately.

Short-term memory

It is best to assess short-term memory (B2a) by questioning the resident regarding very recent occurrences and activities. The resident's ability to clearly remember these happenings could indicate that a memory problem does not exist. The inability to remember could signify a cognitive deficit in this area.

The MDS form identifies a five-minute time frame for testing short-term memory to score this item. One suggestion to test the resident's memory is for the assessor to specifically ask the resident to remember an object or concept and then question the resident five minutes later to see whether he or she can recall it.

A high number of residents who are newly cognitively impaired as identified on the MDS assessment does not necessarily mean that quality of care is lacking. If the nursing facility admits many residents who are in the early stages of senile dementia or Alzheimer's disease, or if a unit in the facility is specifically designated for cognitively impaired residents, progression of these diseases is expected. However, if residents develop impairments in cognitive abilities because of lack of sensory stimulation or boredom, it could indicate a quality-of-care issue requiring further investigation.

At a Glance

Domain #4
Cognitive Patterns

Quality Indicators	MDS Items	MDS Codes
7. Incidence of cognitive impairment	B4: Cognitive skills for daily decision-making	1, 2, or 3 (code present on current MDS and not on previous MDS), and;
	B2a: Short-term memory	1 (code present on current MDS and not on previous MDS)

Chapter 7

Elimination and Incontinence Domain

Review of this quality indicator is crucial to determining quality of care. This domain has not only a sentinel event identified but also the largest number of quality indicators associated with it. The four indicators are the following:

- Prevalence of bladder or bowel incontinence
- Prevalence of occasional or frequent bladder or bowel incontinence without a toileting plan
- Prevalence of indwelling catheters
- Prevalence of fecal impaction

Bladder and bowel incontinence is a major concern for long-term care facilities. The geriatric population in nursing homes has a high incidence of incontinence attributable to disease processes, diminished mental capacities, lack of self-esteem, and depression. Whether a facility is adequately staffed may influence incontinence patterns as well. For instance, an inadequate number of nurses on a particular shift may result in more incontinence episodes because there aren't enough nurses to respond in a timely manner to residents' call bells.

Quality indicator 8: Prevalence of bladder or bowel incontinence

Basic information

- **Indicator type:** Quality indicator 8 monitors data only from the most recent MDS assessment (excluding the initial admission assessment) to obtain the extent of incontinence within the nursing facility.
- **Facility percentage:** Surveyors analyze the facility percentage, which is calculated by comparing those residents coded as at least frequently incontinent of either bladder or bowel with all other residents who have a completed MDS assessment. Unlike the majority of the other quality indicators, this indicator's denominator excludes certain residents: those residents who have an indwelling catheter or ostomy or who are comatose. The Related MDS items section of this chapter discusses coding of these items and their influence on the exclusion.
- **Risk adjustment:** Quality indicator 8 is risk adjusted depending on the amount of cognitive impairment or extent of ADL dependence.

Related MDS items

Section H of the MDS assessment—continence in last 14 days—provides the initial primary information about the flagging of quality indicator 8. Specifically, if you code either bowel continence (H1a) or bladder continence (H1b) as follows, the indicator will be present:

- H1a is coded as a 3 or 4
- H1b is coded as a 3 or 4

You can determine the code for these two items by evaluating the frequency of bladder or bowel incontinence, or both, during the previous 14-day period. A score of 3 designates frequent incontinence, which is defined on the MDS as two to three episodes of bowel incontinence per week or daily bladder incontinence with only slight control present. Scoring a resident as a 4 denotes bowel incontinence all (or almost all) of the time or multiple daily episodes of bladder incontinence. Other possible scores for H1a and H1b that do not affect this quality indicator are 0 for continent, 1 for usually continent, and 2 for occasionally incontinent.

Assessing risk

Quality indicator 8 is risk adjusted; therefore, other MDS items contribute to residents' placement within the indicator parameters. Two conditions—severe cognitive impairment or total dependence in mobility activities of daily living (ADL)—place a resident in the high-risk category. You can consider a resident with neither of these conditions to be at low risk for problems with incontinence.

Severe cognitive impairment

CHSRA has identified severe cognitive impairment as the result of the coding of two MDS items: cognitive skills for daily decision making (B4) and short-term memory (B2a). These are the same MDS items used to determine cognitive impairment in quality indicator 3—prevalence of behavioral symptoms affecting others—and quality indicator 7—incidence of cognitive impairment. The scoring of these items leads to the definition of whether the cognitive impairment is severe. The following codes indicate severe impairment:

- B4 is coded a 3
- B2a is coded a 1

Both of the preceding items must be coded as specified for severe cognitive impairment to be present. As discussed in preceding chapters, a resident coded a 0 in cognitive skills for daily decision making is independent, a 1 indicates modified independence, a 2 designates a moderate impairment, and a 3 indicates a severe impairment, which indicates that the resident rarely or never makes appropriate decisions.

Physical functioning and structural problems

The second condition that places a resident in the incontinence high-risk category is the resident's amount of dependence with mobility-related ADLs. Coding of section G—physical functioning and structural problems—determines the potential for this high-risk status. The ADLs designated as mobility ADLs are bed mobility (G1a), transferring (G1b), and locomotion on the unit (G1e). If you code all of these items as follows, the resident is considered to be high risk:

- G1a box A is coded a 4
- G1b box A is coded a 4
- G1e box A is coded a 4

Only box A—ADL self-performance—is considered for this risk adjustment. Box B—ADL support provided—does not influence this quality indicator. The range of codes that can be entered in box A for these ADLs are 0 (independent), 1 (supervision), 2 (limited assistance), 3 (extensive assistance), 4 (total dependence), or 8 (the activity did not occur). Residents will be placed in the high-risk category only if you code that they were totally dependent for the ADLs of bed mobility, transferring, and locomotion on the unit.

If neither severe cognitive impairment nor total mobility ADL dependence is present, the resident is placed in the low-risk category for bladder or bowel incontinence.

Exclusion of residents

The final group of MDS items that affects quality indicator 8 pertains to the residents who are excluded from the denominator of the facility percentage. The majority of the prevalence quality indicators includes all residents with a current MDS assessment in the denominator; however, this quality indicator excludes those residents who are coded specifically in one of three categories: comatose (B1), indwelling catheter (H3d), and ostomy (H3i). If you code any one of these items as follows, the resident will be excluded from the denominator of the facility percentage:

- B1 is coded a 1
- H3d is checked
- H3i is checked

B1 indicates whether a resident is in a coma. A score of 0 means not comatose, and a score of 1 means comatose. You should check the appropriate item in section H—indwelling catheter or ostomy—if either is present.

MDS assessment and coding

Many items can influence quality indicator 8 in various ways. Items on the MDS can designate a resident as having bowel or bladder incontinence, further classify a resident as high-risk or low-risk, or exclude a resident from the pool of residents in the denominator.

Continence

You should code the continence of a resident in section H1 of the MDS. This section is another exception to the seven-day assessment rule: All responses pertain to the previous 14-day, or two-week, period. Additionally, the MDS specifically states that the coding must include the resident's performance over all shifts. Frequently, a resident who is continent during the day when awake or more alert might have episodes of incontinence during nighttime hours. When assessing this area of a resident's health status, it is important to elicit information from staff on all shifts who may have information about the resident's continence status. Daily documentation in the chart also provides needed input for this assessment.

Assessment of the resident's continence status should also include a direct conversation with the resident and his or her family members, if possible. Assessors should consider the sensitive nature of this topic and preserve the resident's dignity in discussing it. A nursing home resident may deny incontinence because of embarrassment. Family members and astute staff should be questioned if a discrepancy exists between what the resident reports and the actual condition.

Code both bladder and bowel incontinence based on the frequency of the incontinent episodes during the 14-day assessment period. The coding ranges from complete control of elimination to incontinence of both bowel and bladder. Note that a resident who has an indwelling catheter or an ostomy, and does not have any leakage, is considered continent. In other words, even if an indwelling catheter/ostomy is inserted to prevent or control incontinence, and the resident would be incontinent without the catheter or ostomy, the resident would now be considered continent.

Each of the codes for section H1 pertains to both bladder and bowel incontinence; however, the codes do not always designate the same frequency of each type of incontinence. As an example, a score of 3 (frequently incontinent) means that a resident was daily incontinent of bladder but only incontinent of bowel two to three times per week. Therefore, rather than using the same code for both bladder and bowel functions, assessors should use separate codes to reflect the frequency of bladder and bowel functions.

Continence programs

You should also consider continence programs when coding section H1. If a resident would be incontinent without intervention but is now continent because of a toileting program, you should still code the resident as continent. Scoring in this area reflects the current 14-day continence status of the resident rather than the anticipated status without the use of a continence program.

Cognitive skills for daily decision making

The risk adjustment of severe cognitive impairment for quality indicator 8 results in the review of extra MDS items to determine the further classification of residents. Cognitive skills for daily decision making (B4) and short-term memory (B2a) are the additional MDS items used to determine cognitive impairment for quality indicator 3—prevalence of behavioral symptoms affecting others—and quality indicator 7—incidence of cognitive impairment. To review, item B4 addresses the resident's ability to make decisions within his or her environment during the seven-day assessment period. Staff members assessing for this item should question the resident directly about his or her perceived abilities and also consult with other staff members regarding the amount of intervention required. If a resident has cognitive loss to the degree that he or she cannot make rational decisions about daily activities, this deficit, combined with short-term memory loss, would indicate severe cognitive impairment.

Memory loss

Memory loss can be tested with structured memory tests or by questioning the resident about recent happenings. If the resident cannot accurately remember recent activities, the caretaker should code the resident as having a short-term memory problem on the MDS.

Activities of daily living

The second variable for the determination of risk adjustment is the amount of resident dependence with mobility ADLs as coded in section G of the MDS. Column A of section G, self-performance, pertains to the resident's performance of the specified ADLs during all shifts for the seven-day assessment period. Therefore, consult with staff members on all shifts when determining this coding because a resident's ability to perform ADLs can vary greatly depending on the time of day. A resident who is mobile during the morning and early afternoon hours might become more dependent on staff assistance during the evening. Questioning the resident can help determine the extent of staff intervention required.

The directions for coding the ADL section of the MDS are explicit and should be read carefully. You should carefully determine the actual amount of oversight, encouragement, and/or weight-bearing support needed, document the assistance, and then score according to the parameters for each ADL as identified on the MDS.

The mobility ADLs affecting risk adjustment for quality indicator 8 are bed mobility, transferring, and locomotion on the unit. Do not consider locomotion off the unit (G1f) for quality indicator 8. Bed mobility assesses the ability of the resident to move while in bed, position self, and turn from side to side. Transferring assesses the resident's capability to transfer between bed, chair (including a wheelchair), and a standing position. Transfers to and from the toilet are not included in this item. Item G1i addresses toilet transferring. Locomotion on the unit assesses the resident's ability to move in the room and the corridor outside the room. This item also includes the resident's ability to perform locomotion when in a wheelchair or with an assistive device, such as a cane or walker. The use of these devices should not change the level of the coding for this item. For example, a resident who uses a wheelchair and can move about the unit independently once in the wheelchair would be scored a 0, designating that no help or oversight is required.

If you code a resident a 4, total dependence, in all three of these areas of mobility, he or she should be assigned to the high-risk category. Total dependence means that the resident did not participate at all in the activity; staff members were required to perform the entire ADL. If a resident is able to initiate and perform even a small portion of the designated activity, the coding should reflect this resident's involvement; he or she should not be considered totally dependent.

Exclusion of residents

You must consider the proper assessment and coding of three other MDS items that relate to the denominator exclusion for quality indicator 8. Because this quality indicator measures the presence of bowel or bladder incontinence in the nursing facility, those residents who do not have the potential to be incontinent or could not have incontinence managed are excluded. Only residents who could possibly develop a problem with incontinence are considered when determining the facility percentage. Therefore, the three underlying conditions that exclude residents from possible incontinence or incontinence management are the presence of a coma (B1), indwelling catheter (H3d), or ostomy (H3i). A comatose resident cannot indicate the need for toileting or have incontinent episodes decreased through a toileting plan. As is indicated in section H of the MDS, residents with a nonleaking urinary catheter or ostomy are considered continent; this status would only change if the appliance was removed or began to leak. Because the potential to develop incontinence or have incontinence managed is unlikely for residents with these three qualifiers, they are excluded from the denominator of the facility percentage.

Nursing homes with a high percentage of residents with bladder or bowel incontinence warrant regulatory examination to determine the reasons for the incontinence and whether an incontinence management program is in place. A large number of incontinent residents in a nursing facility does not necessarily reflect poor quality care. The type and primary diagnoses of these residents could indicate why the incontinence exists. Proper management and evaluation of this incontinence show recognition and awareness of the condition and demonstrate measures are in place to maintain the highest possible quality existence for all residents. The next quality indicator pertains to incontinence management.

Quality indicator 9: Prevalence of occasional or frequent bladder or bowel incontinence without a toileting plan

Basic information

- **Indicator type:** Quality indicator 9 is a prevalence indicator using data only from the most recently completed MDS assessment (excluding the admission assessment).

- **Facility percentage:** Surveyors analyze the facility percentage, which is calculated by comparing those residents without a coded toileting plan on the current MDS with those residents who were coded as being either frequently or occasionally incontinent of bladder or bowel on the current MDS.

As explained in the discussion of quality indicator 8, the denominator used to arrive at the facility percentage is not based on all residents in the nursing home with a completed MDS. Because this indicator only examines residents who are occasionally or frequently incontinent, only these incontinent residents should be included in the denominator.

- **Risk adjustment:** Quality indicator 9 is not risk adjusted.

Related MDS items

Section H—continence in the last 14 days—provides all the information needed for determining the presence or lack of perceived quality for quality indicator 9. Two items on the MDS pertain to toileting plans: any scheduled toileting plan (H3a) and bladder retraining program (H3b). These items are coded according to whether the programs are in place and being used for a resident. If either or both programs are present, the appropriate item (or items) is checked. If the plans are not being used, the boxes are left blank. This quality indicator could be flagged if either of the items are coded as follows:

- H3a is not checked
- H3b is not checked

You do not need to check both items to indicate that a toileting plan is present. Even checking only one item and leaving the other blank indicates a toileting program is in place and that staff are attempting to manage incontinence. Once again, this section is an exception to the seven-day assessment period rule. When completing the preceding two items, the previous 14 days must be considered.

If a resident is flagged for quality indicator 9, this indicates that not only is a toileting program not in place but the resident is also either frequently or occasionally incontinent of bladder or bowel. The following MDS items, coded as below, would indicate occasional or frequent incontinence:

- H1a is coded a 2 or 3
- H1b is coded a 2 or 3

As with the toileting program, both of these items do not need to be coded for the resident to be considered either occasionally incontinent, a score of 2, or frequently incontinent, a score of 3. If you score either bowel continence (H1a) or bladder continence (H1b) as a 2 or 3, the resident is considered in the denominator for the facility percentage, which could cause this indicator to flag. A 14-day period for incontinence is reviewed to determine the proper scoring for these items.

MDS assessment and coding

When coding and assessing a scheduled toileting plan (H3a) and bladder retraining program (H3b), it is important to understand the definitions of these two items. Assessors often are reluctant to code for these programs because they think that a structured, elaborate plan must be in place. Failure to accurately code these items could result in an artificially high number of incontinent residents and could potentially flag this indicator.

Scheduled toileting plan

A scheduled toileting plan is defined as a program used during the day where staff members either take the resident to the toilet or remind the resident to go to the bathroom. The key concept with this plan is that the toileting or prompting is conducted at a set schedule throughout the day. For example, if a resident is always taken to the bathroom before and after all meals, and this plan is documented, item H3a could be checked. As long as a schedule is maintained, the program is considered a toileting plan for managing incontinence. Both bladder and bowel incontinence can be managed with this type of plan.

Bladder retraining program

A bladder retraining program differs from a scheduled toileting plan by placing more emphasis on the resident consciously waiting to urinate, thereby training the bladder to hold urine and, in theory, decreasing the number of episodes of incontinence. This type of program is usually more successful with residents who are cognitively aware and capable of delaying voiding. If such a program is being used, code it on the MDS in item H3b.

To accurately code for either of the preceding two programs, facility staff must verify documentation of these plans. The previous 14 days should be assessed for toileting programs that are documented in the nurse's notes, flow sheets, treatment records, and nursing care plan. Nursing assistants can also provide valuable information regarding toileting programs used and their success or failure.

Residents who are occasionally or frequently incontinent are included in the denominator for the facility percentage determination and potential flagging of this quality indicator. Assessors should exclude those residents who are continent or totally incontinent. It is important to accurately code this information to correctly assign the residents. For bowel continence (H1a), code a resident a 2 (occasionally incontinent) if the bowel incontinence occurs only once a week, or a 3 (frequently incontinent) if the bowel incontinence occurs two to three times per week. Code bladder continence (H1b) a 2 (occasionally incontinent) if the episodes of incontinence occur two or more times per week but not every day, or a 3 (frequently incontinent) if the resident is incontinent on a daily basis but still has some control over bladder elimination.

When coding for incontinence, the assessment period includes the 14 days up to and including the assessment reference date of the MDS. The resident's elimination status over that two-week period should be monitored and appropriately coded. Each of the codes for section H1 includes parameters for both bowel and bladder continence for each value. When coding this section, assessors must read these parameters carefully to determine the proper code for each type of incontinence. Chart documentation, conversations with staff members on all shifts, as well as the resident and family members will help assessors determine the correct response.

A high prevalence of incontinence without toileting plans in place could warrant investigation by regulatory agencies to determine whether a problem with care exists. Frequently, nurse assessors might undercode the number of toileting programs in a nursing home, either because they don't realize that a program exists or because they don't consider the less structured programs. If the incidence of incontinence is indeed high and efforts to prevent this incontinence are not being used, surveyors could question quality of care.

Quality indicator 10: Prevalence of indwelling catheters

Basic information

- **Indicator type:** Quality indicator 10, the third quality indicator included in the elimination/incontinence domain, addresses the use of indwelling catheters in the nursing facility. Surveyors use only the information generated from the most recent MDS assessment submitted (excluding the initial admission assessment) to determine this prevalence.

- **Facility percentage:** Surveyors analyze the facility percentage, which is obtained by comparing those residents who have an indwelling catheter with all other residents in the nursing home with a completed MDS assessment.

- **Risk adjustment:** Quality indicator 10 is not risk adjusted.

Related MDS item

Only data from one item on the MDS contribute to the determination of the flagging of quality indicator 10: indwelling catheter (H3d). Section H of the MDS—continence in last 14 days—is another exception to the usual seven-day assessment period. The two-week period up to and including the assessment reference date of the MDS should be reviewed to determine whether an indwelling catheter is present. The MDS guidelines define an indwelling catheter as those catheters inserted through the urethra into the bladder or inserted through a suprapubic incisional site directly into the bladder. An external condom catheter or intermittent catheterization are not included in this definition. If an indwelling catheter is present, check item H3d on the MDS; if no indwelling catheter is present, leave item H3d blank.

MDS assessment and coding

Presence or absence of indwelling catheter

The assessment of the presence or absence of an indwelling catheter is relatively straightforward. As discussed, a 14-day assessment period should be used. Documentation in the medical record indicates whether a resident has an indwelling catheter; direct observation and conversation with the resident and staff members will confirm this. The lack of a urinary collection device, such as a drainage bag, does not necessarily mean that a catheter is not being used. A leg bag or other means of discrete urinary collection that is not visible could be worn by the resident.

The use of indwelling catheters is an important determinant of quality of care within a nursing home. If a high percentage of residents have indwelling catheters, questions might be raised about whether these catheters are essential or if their insertion was due to routine physician orders or staff convenience. Review may determine that some of the indwelling catheters could be removed, thereby decreasing the risk of infection or urethral injury. Conversely, the catheters might be necessary for adequate bladder elimination status.

Quality indicator 11: Prevalence of fecal impaction

Basic information

- **Indicator type:** Quality indicator 11 is the final indicator included under the elimination/incontinence domain and could be considered the most important in this area. Fecal impaction is the first of three designated sentinel events. A sentinel event is so serious that even the presence of one resident with this condition causes great concern about quality of care. The indicator is a prevalence indicator, meaning that data from only the most recent MDS assessment (excluding the initial admission assessment) are used.

- **Facility percentage:** Surveyors analyze the facility percentage, which is determined by comparing those residents who have a coded fecal impaction with all residents in the facility with a completed MDS assessment.

- **Risk adjustment:** Quality indicator 11 is not risk adjusted.

Related MDS item

Only one MDS item—fecal impaction (H2d)—affects the possible flagging of this indicator. Section H contains the primary data used for the determination of quality in this domain. As discussed previously, staff should assess all items in section H by reviewing a 14-day assessment period; therefore, the presence or absence of a fecal impaction must be assessed by reviewing these 14 days.

MDS assessment and coding

Fecal impaction

When determining whether a resident has fecal impaction, distinguish between constipation and impaction. Constipation is defined as two or fewer bowel movements per week or straining more than one of four times when moving the bowels. Impaction is the occurrence of feces so firmly and tightly packed together so as to be immovable. However, a resident might have a fecal impaction and still be able to have very small bowel movements.

Because this quality indicator is a sentinel event, it is critical that you properly assess and code item H2d. If a resident is diagnosed with a fecal impaction, first determine whether this impaction was present during the 14-day assessment period. If the impaction occurred before this time, it would not be coded. If a resident is constipated, this does not automatically mean that a fecal impaction is present.

Documentation in the medical record will assist with the coding for fecal impactions, as will a digital rectal examination. Nursing assistants from all shifts should be questioned about bowel elimination status, and input from the resident is important.

The presence of only one resident coded as having a fecal impaction will result in a review of that individual to determine the circumstances leading up to this condition. In the majority of residents, fecal impaction is preventable through adequate fluid intake, proper diet, and judicious use of laxatives. Therefore, fecal impaction in nursing home residents may indicate a lower quality of care. Further investigation would reveal whether the impaction could have been prevented or whether the care (or lack of care) provided could have contributed to the condition. It is vital to accurately determine whether fecal impaction exists to ensure that you correctly code this portion of the MDS.

At a Glance

Domain #5
Elimination/Incontinence

Quality Indicators	MDS Items	MDS Codes
8. Prevalence of bladder or bowel incontinence	H1b: Bladder continence	3 or 4, or;
	H1a: Bowel continence	3 or 4
Exclusion of residents for QI #8	B1: Comatose	1, or;
	H3d: Indwelling catheter	Box is checked, or;
	H3i: Ostomy present	Box is checked
High risk for QI #8	B4: Cognitive skills for daily decision making	3, and;
	B2a: Short-term memory	1
	OR	
	G1a Box A: Bed mobility self-performance	4, and;

Domain #5 (cont.)

Quality Indicators	MDS Items	MDS Codes
See previous page	G1b Box A: Transfer self-performance	4, and;
	G1e Box A: Locomotion on unit self-performance	4
Low risk for QI #8: all other residents not classified as high risk	N/A	N/A
9. Prevalence of occasional or frequent bladder or bowel incontinence without a toileting plan	H3a: Any scheduled toileting plan	Box is not checked, and;
	H3b: Bladder retraining program	Box is not checked
	AND	
	H1b: Bladder continence	2 or 3, or;
	H1a: Bowel continence	2 or 3

Domain #5 (cont.)		
Quality Indicators	**MDS Items**	**MDS Codes**
10. Prevalence of indwelling catheters	H3d: Indwelling catheter	Box is checked
11. Prevalence of fecal impaction	H2d: Fecal impaction	Box is checked

Chapter 8

Infection Control Domain

The prevention and control of infections are extremely important in the long-term care (LTC) environment. An infection easily resolved in younger patients may be life-threatening to elderly nursing home residents because of their compromised medical status and decreased resistance to disease. Nursing home staff must always practice good infection control, ranging from proper hand washing to isolation techniques, depending on the type of organism and the method of transmission. Infections acquired in the LTC facility (facility-acquired infections) should be prevented as much as possible; a low rate of this kind of infection transmission could indicate quality care. Although many types of infections can be present in nursing homes, only one type of infection is included in the infection control domain: the presence of urinary tract infections.

Quality indicator 12: Prevalence of urinary tract infections

Basic information

- **Indicator type:** Quality indicator 12, the sole indicator in the infection control domain, obtains its data from the most recent MDS assessment (excluding the initial admission assessment).

- **Facility percentage:** Surveyors analyze the facility percentage, which is calculated by comparing the number of residents with a urinary tract infection coded on the current MDS with all other residents who have a completed MDS assessment.

- **Risk adjustment:** Quality indicator 12 is not risk adjusted.

Related MDS item

Only one MDS item provides data for this infection control indicator: urinary tract infection in the last 30 days (I2j). Once again, the usual seven-day assessment period is not used; the assessment must include a review for urinary tract infections during a 30-day time period. It is important to consider that a urinary tract infection occurring exactly one month before the assessment date might not be within this 30-day time frame. The MDS assessor should carefully count the number of days to determine how to code this item. If a urinary tract infection was present during the preceding described time period, the assessor checks item I2j. If no urinary tract infection occurred, item I2j remains blank.

MDS assessment and coding

Urinary tract infections

Urinary tract infections in the elderly may be exhibited in various ways; therefore, astute observation and assessment are needed. Assessors should code both chronic and acute urinary tract infections if signs and symptoms are present. The alert, oriented resident might complain about burning during urination or lower back pain, whereas a disoriented resident might only exhibit increased confusion, agitation, or an elevated temperature.

It is important that supporting laboratory results are present to indicate whether a urinary tract infection exists. If the preceding evidence is not available, accurately determining the presence of a urinary tract infection can be difficult. Code urinary tract infections if the resident's symptoms indicate one is present, you have a physician's working diagnosis, and you are waiting for laboratory results. If laboratory results later show that the resident did not have a urinary tract infection, complete a correction to that MDS.

Urinary tract infections diagnosed and resolved before the assessment period should not be coded in item I2j; consider only urinary tract infections occurring within the previous 30 days. If a resident has an active diagnosis of recurrent urinary tract infections but did not experience one during the assessment period, this diagnosis is entered in other current or more detailed diagnoses and ICD-9 codes (I3).

Only symptomatic, documented urinary tract infections must be coded in I2j. This information may be obtained from the medical record—specifically, documentation in physician's progress notes, nurse's notes, and laboratory reports. Cognitively aware residents can also provide information as to whether they have a urinary tract infection, and these reports of infections should be confirmed with the supporting documentation.

A large number of residents with urinary tract infections might indicate a quality of care problem. Inadequate infection control techniques, lack of sufficient fluid intake, improper catheter insertion, or presence of facility-acquired infections are just a few reasons why an increased number of urinary tract infections could occur. Further clarification and investigation will help determine whether the infections were preventable or whether a quality-care issue is evident.

At a Glance

Domain #6
Infection Control

Quality Indicators	MDS Items	MDS Codes
12. Prevalence of urinary tract infections	I2j: Urinary tract infection in last 30 days	Box is checked

Chapter 9

Nutrition and Eating Domain

The importance of adequate nutrition and fluid intake for the predominantly older population of nursing homes cannot be overstated. Because of the compromised physiologic status of many elderly residents, proper nutrition is essential, contributing to increased quality of life and inhibiting further progression of disease processes. Many nutritional issues can arise during regulatory reviews, including a resident's appetite and weight and even presentation of meals. This domain considers three aspects of nutrition:

- Prevalence of weight loss
- Prevalence of tube feedings
- Prevalence of dehydration

The seriousness of dehydration distinguishes it as the second of three sentinel events.

Quality indicator 13: Prevalence of weight loss

Basic information

- **Indicator type:** Quality indicator 13, the first indicator in the nutrition and eating domain, is a prevalence indicator that considers data from only the most recently completed MDS assessment (excluding the initial admission assessment).

- **Facility percentage:** Surveyors analyze the facility percentage, which is calculated by comparing those residents who have a specific amount of weight loss—5% or more in the past 30 days, or 10% or more in the past 180 days—to all residents with a completed MDS assessment.
- **Risk adjustment:** Quality indicator 13 is not risk adjusted.

Relevant MDS item

Only one MDS item—weight change (K3)—contributes data to the potential flagging of quality indicator 13. Specifically, weight loss (K3a) is the only item from this section used for the data. A weight gain is not considered in this quality indicator. Score weight loss a 1 for yes if either of the following two conditions is met:

- Weight loss is 5% or more within the previous 30 days
- Weight loss is 10% or more within the previous 180 days

Only one of the two preceding scenarios needs to occur for staff to code a significant weight loss. According to these parameters, if neither of the two conditions applies, a significant weight loss has not occurred and you should score item K3a a 0.

Once again, an exception to the usual seven-day assessment period is used. A 30-day period for the 5% weight loss and a 180-day period for the 10% weight loss must be reviewed and assessed. It is important to count actual days when performing this assessment rather than just considering a one-month or six-month time period. For example, a date exactly six months before the assessment reference date would be more than 180 days. Depending on the number of days in the calendar month being reviewed, a 30-day look-back period could be more or less than exactly one calendar month.

MDS assessment and coding

Weight loss

Make two primary considerations when coding item K3a: the accuracy of the weight measurement and the accuracy of the calculation of the weight change. When weighing a resident follow the same procedure for each measurement to obtain comparable weights. Depending on the policy of the facility, staff must determine what time of day the weight should be taken and whether weighing should occur before a meal. You should weigh a resident in the same type of clothing at all times and without shoes (or per facility policy). If you use a wheelchair scale, the weight of the wheelchair must be accurately recorded and subtracted from the total weight of the wheelchair plus the resident. You should also measure weight after a resident has voided, as this could alter the resident's weight by several pounds. Do not round residents' weights.

Whether a scale is stationary or is moved when used for weights, recalibration of the scale is critical for correct weight measurements. If possible, staff should use the same scale for every weighing to obtain accurate comparisons between current and previous weights. Using different scales could lead to an artificial weight change due only to the different type of equipment used.

Staff members responsible for weighing residents should receive adequate training in the preceding procedures. If a weight appears to be significantly different from a previous weight, reweighing should be done to determine the accuracy of the new weight.

Calculating the percentage of weight loss for item K3a can be confusing. Two calculations should be considered when completing this assessment: the percentage weight change during the previous 30 days and the percentage weight change during the previous 180 days. The most current weight should be used to determine the percentage weight loss for both time periods. Before item K3a can be completed, both calculations must be precise, as a weight change might be above the percentage threshold for one time period and not for the other.

To determine whether a 5% or more weight loss has occurred, subtract the most recent weight from the weight from 30 days ago. Then divide this number by the weight from 30 days ago and multiply it by 100 to obtain the percentage weight change. If this percentage equals five or more, a significant weight loss has occurred.

Determining whether a 10% or more weight loss occurred is calculated similarly: Subtract the current weight from the weight obtained 180 days ago. Divide this number by the weight from 180 days ago and then multiply by 100. If this percentage equals 10 or higher, a significant weight loss has occurred.

When counting the number of days (30 or 180) to determine weight loss, the assessment reference date of the MDS is the final day in the assessment time period. For example, an MDS with an assessment reference date of the first day of a calendar month only includes data from the 30 days or 180 days before that assessment date. Do not consider weights obtained outside those time frames when calculating the weight change percentages.

Nursing home staff should document information about the resident's weight in the clinical chart. If a resident is newly admitted to the nursing facility and current records are not available going back 30 or 180 days, documentation from a prior healthcare facility or consultation with the physician and family members could yield the information to accurately determine whether any weight loss has occurred.

A high percentage of residents with weight loss could indicate a problem with the nutritional status of residents at a nursing home. Further investigation would reveal whether the weight loss was unavoidable, as in cases of deteriorating medical conditions such as cancer or other terminal illnesses. Other reasons for weight loss include a resident's dislike of foods offered, inadequate staffing patterns, or untreated resident depression. That determination must be made to decide whether the facility should institute quality improvement measures.

Quality indicator 14: Prevalence of tube feeding

Basic information

- **Indicator type:** Quality indicator 14, the second indicator in this domain, is also a prevalence indicator using information about tube feedings from the most recently completed MDS (excluding the initial admission assessment).

- **Facility percentage:** Surveyors analyze the facility percentage, which is calculated by comparing all residents indicated as having tube feedings with all residents who have a completed MDS assessment.

- **Risk adjustment:** Quality indicator 14 is not risk adjusted.

Related MDS item

Only one MDS item affects the flagging of quality indicator 14: feeding tube (K5b). The assessment period used to determine the presence or absence of a feeding tube is the usual seven-day time frame with the assessment reference date being the final day in the time period. If a feeding tube is present during this seven-day period, check item K5b. This item remains blank if no feeding tube is present.

MDS assessment and coding

Feeding tube

Determining whether a resident has a feeding tube can be done by observation of the resident and review of the clinical record. Types of feeding tubes are defined in the MDS completion manual as nasogastric, gastrostomy, jejunostomy, and percutaneous endoscopic gastrostomy (PEG) tubes.

Note that the mere presence of a feeding tube should prompt staff to check this item. Even if the tube was not used during the seven-day assessment period as a route to deliver food, fluids, or medications, check item K5b. The next item in section K, item K6, assesses the amount of calories and fluid administered to a resident via a feeding tube. This item, however, does not have any effect on this quality indicator. Therefore, if a feeding tube is no longer used but is still present, consult with the physician to determine whether the feeding tube is still required.

Regulatory agencies would scrutinize a nursing home with a high percentage of feeding tubes to determine the reason for the use of these tubes. The facility might specialize in the care of residents whose conditions require feeding tubes, such as residents unable to swallow due to cerebrovascular accidents or coma. Conversely, the nursing home might use feeding tubes more frequently than expected because of oral feeding difficulties. Further investigation should reveal why a high number of feeding tubes is present.

Quality indicator 15: Prevalence of dehydration

Basic information

- **Indicator type:** Quality indicator 15, the final indicator in this domain, is also a prevalence indicator. Information from the most recently completed MDS assessment (excluding the initial admission assessment) determines whether this indicator is flagged. Dehydration is one of three sentinel events and is so serious that even if a facility only has one dehydrated resident, regulatory agencies will extensively study and review the case. Surveyors will scrutinize the clinical record to determine why the dehydration occurred and whether it could have been prevented. Therefore, accurate coding of this area on the MDS is essential.

- **Facility percentage:** Surveyors analyze the facility percentage, which is calculated by considering all residents identified as having dehydration compared with all residents with a completed MDS assessment.

- **Risk adjustment:** No risk adjustment is used with quality indicator 15.

Related MDS items

Dehydration is marked in one of two places on the MDS. The first item to consider is dehydrated—output exceeds input (J1c). You should use a seven-day assessment period to determine the response for this item. If dehydration is present, check the item; if no dehydration exists, the item is left blank.

The second area of the MDS in which dehydration could be coded is other current or more detailed diagnoses and ICD-9 codes (I3). A diagnosis code of 276.5 (volume depletion) triggers this quality indicator even if dehydration is not checked in item J1c. Diagnosis codes entered in I3 relate to the resident's current medical status and do not include old, inactive diagnoses.

MDS assessment and coding

Code dehydration in item J1c if at least two of the following conditions are present:

- The resident ingests less than the recommended 1,500 mL of fluids daily.
- The resident has actual clinical indicators of dehydration.
- The resident's loss of fluids is greater than the amount of fluids ingested.

If none or only one of the preceding three indicators is present, do not code dehydration in item J1c.

In reviewing these three indicators, fluid in both food and liquids must be considered to determine whether the resident is usually taking in 1,500 mL of fluid. Clinical indicators of dehydration include a dry tongue and mouth, decreased production of urine, sunken eyes, decreased skin turgor, confusion, and a rapid or weak heartbeat. Fluid loss greater than fluid ingestion can occur with extensive bleeding, diuretic therapy, vomiting and diarrhea, or a fever, which can cause the resident to perspire. The supporting documentation in a resident's chart, in addition to conversations with the resident and staff, will help determine whether these conditions are present.

Consider all of the preceding descriptions of the indicators of dehydration before coding item J1c. Although the MDS form lists the actual description of only one of the preceding three scenarios—output exceeds input—two of the three conditions must be present for dehydration to be coded.

Additionally, only a seven-day assessment period is used for this section of the MDS. If dehydration occurred before the assessment period, do not code it. Even if a resident has a physician diagnosis of dehydration from a previous hospital stay, code the dehydration only if two of the preceding three conditions were present during the assessment period. If the resident has a current diagnosis of dehydration that pertains to the resident's medical status, enter the ICD-9 code of 276.5 in item I3. You should not include an old, resolved, or inactive diagnosis of dehydration in this section.

Because dehydration is considered a sentinel event, one resident with this condition would cause surveyors to question whether quality care is being provided. Both accurate assessment and documentation of care provided to alleviate the dehydration are crucial. If a nursing home is not performing proper identification, implementation of the care plan, and evaluation of results, regulatory agencies could question whether quality care is present.

At a Glance

Domain #7

Nutrition/Eating

Quality Indicators	MDS Items	MDS Codes
13. Prevalence of weight loss	K3a: Weight change-weight loss	1
14. Prevalence of tube feeding	K5b: Feeding tube	Box is checked
15. Prevalence of dehydration	J1c: Dehydrated (output exceeds input)	Box is checked, or;
	I3: Other current or more detailed diagnoses and ICD-9 codes	Diagnosis ICD-9 code is 276.5

Chapter 10

Physical Functioning Domain

The ability to move freely and participate in daily events is important for everyone. The effects of aging diminish the capacity of many elderly nursing home residents to physically move as they desire. This disability leads to other problems such as depression, exacerbation of current conditions, and development of new diseases related to immobility. This domain includes three quality indicators pertaining to physical functioning:

- Prevalence of bedfast residents
- Incidence of a decline in late-loss ADLs
- Incidence of decline in range of motion (ROM)

All of these indicators are important in determining the nursing home resident's ability to physically function as normally as possible.

Quality indicator 16: Prevalence of bedfast residents

Basic information

- **Indicator type:** Quality indicator 16, the first quality indicator in the physical functioning domain, uses data obtained from the most recently completed MDS assessment to determine the percentage of residents who are bedfast.

- **Facility percentage:** Surveyors analyze the facility percentage, which is calculated by comparing those residents who are coded as being bedfast with all other residents in the nursing center who have a completed MDS assessment.
- **Risk adjustment:** Quality indicator 16 is not risk adjusted.

Related MDS item

Only one MDS item can cause this quality indicator to flag. In the modes of transfer portion of the physical functioning and structural problems section, bedfast all or most of the time (G6a) provides the required information. You should use a seven-day assessment period to determine whether a resident is bedfast. To perform an accurate assessment of this area, the definition of bedfast must be clarified.

MDS assessment and coding

Bedfast all or most of the time

The MDS manual provides a specific definition of what constitutes a bedfast resident. If the following two conditions are present, you should check this item:

- The resident is in bed or in a recliner in his or her room for at least 22 hours per day.
- The preceding occurs on at least four of the seven days that constitute the assessment period.

Both of these conditions must be met for item G6a to be checked. For example, if the resident is in bed at least 22 hours per day, but only on three days during the assessment period, do not check the item.

The MDS completion directions also refer to residents who are able to go to the bathroom or use a commode but otherwise are in bed. If the preceding two conditions still apply, you should consider the resident bedfast.

Note that if the resident is outside of his or her room for more than two hours per day, even if in a reclining chair, you should not code the resident as bedfast. For example, a resident who is placed in a reclining geri-chair, then wheeled to a location such as a sitting room or area near a nursing station, is no longer bedfast if the resident is in the chair outside of his or her room for more than two hours daily. If, however, that same resident is placed in a reclining geri-chair, but remains in his or her room, he or she should be coded as bedfast.

When you perform the assessment for this item, chart documentation and direct observation should provide the necessary information. Because of their amount of hands-on care and direct observation of the resident, nursing assistants can provide valuable input about the specific time parameters used to determine bedfastness.

Regulatory agencies will scrutinize nursing centers with a high percentage of bedfast residents to determine the reasons for the high number. A facility may admit and care for many critical, unstable, or terminal residents who are unable to be out of bed. On the other hand, if it is determined that residents remained in bed due to lack of sufficient staff, a quality of care issue is present and could result in regulatory sanctions.

Quality indicator 17: Incidence of decline in late-loss activities of daily living

Basic information

- **Indicator type:** Quality indicator 17, the second quality indicator in the physical functioning domain, is an incidence indicator. A change over time is measured by using data obtained from the most recent MDS assessment (excluding the initial admission assessment) compared to the prior MDS completed. Changes in coding of ADL-related items between these two MDSs are reviewed for any noted decline in ADL status.

- **Facility percentage:** Surveyors analyze the facility percentage, which is calculated by comparing those residents who have had a specific numerically coded decline over two MDS assessments in the self-performance ability of late-loss ADLs with all other residents who have two completed MDS assessments. An exclusion is used in figuring the denominator for this percentage: Residents who already are totally dependent or comatose and cannot decline any further in ADL status are not included in the denominator for the facility percentage.

- **Risk adjustment:** Quality indicator 17 is not risk adjusted.

Related MDS items

Section G—physical functioning and structural problems—provides the majority of the information for this quality indicator. Four ADLs have been defined as late-loss ADLs, meaning ADLs that a resident tends to be capable of performing the longest, even with a declining physical condition. Bed mobility (G1a), transferring (G1b), eating (G1h), and toileting (G1i) are designated as late-loss ADLs. The remaining ADLs in section G (walking, locomotion, dressing, personal hygiene, and bathing) are more complex, and the resident's ability to perform these ADLs tends to decrease earlier than the designated late-loss ADLs.

Similar to the risk-adjustment ADL items in quality indicator 8 (bladder or bowel incontinence), only the ADL self-performance column, box A, provides the required data for this indicator. The ADL support-provided column, box B, is not used. ADL self-performance coding depends on the level of ADL assistance required, ranging from a score of 0 for independent to a score of 4 for totally dependent. Use a score of 8 to designate that the activity did not occur.

What causes the indicator to flag?

For this indicator to flag, one of two ADL declines must be present. The numerical declines are a

- one-level decline in two or more late-loss ADLs
- two-level decline in one or more late-loss ADLs

Only one of the preceding scenarios must be present for potential flagging. Each numerical code of bed mobility, transferring, eating, and toileting that appears in box A is considered to be a level. When comparing two MDS forms, if a level on the most recent MDS is scored at a higher number than the previous MDS, a decline in that ADL has occurred. For example, if staff coded transferring as a 1 (supervision) on the prior MDS but now code it a 2 (limited assistance) on the current MDS, a one-level decline occurred. If the self-performance code on the current MDS is a 3 (extensive assistance), a two-level decline occurred. CHSRA has determined that a score of 8 (activity did not occur) is treated as no data present for that ADL because if the ADL did not occur in the first place, it cannot decline further.

Exclusion of residents

The exclusion of certain residents from the denominator of the facility percentage results in the use of other MDS items for this indicator. All 10 ADLs listed in section G1 (items G1a–j box A) are considered when excluding residents. If all 10 items on the prior MDS are coded a 4 (total dependence) or an 8 (activity did not occur), no further decline in ADL self-performance is possible. Residents who are designated as comatose (item B1 is scored a 1) are also excluded. The total dependence in both ADL status and coma do not need to occur; if only one of the preceding two situations exists, the resident is excluded from the facility percentage.

MDS assessment and coding

Section G1—physical functioning and structural problems—can cause difficulties for MDS assessors. Note that two distinct types of ADL assistance are measured for each identified ADL: the resident's self-performance (box A) and the amount of support provided (box B). Coding for each of these boxes requires the assessment period to be the last seven days ending with the assessment reference date of the MDS. You should not assess the ADL status before that time period. Assessors tend to code this section according to the perceived long-term status of the resident for each ADL, but a dramatic change during the seven-day assessment period could occur, which the coding should reflect.

Resident's self-performance

Assessors can measure the resident's ADL self-performance, excluding setup, by entering the corresponding status code over all shifts. Because a resident's ability to perform a specific ADL during the course of the day and night might vary significantly, consult with staff on all shifts to determine the proper coding. Because of the direct care they give and the amount of time they spend with the resident, nursing assistants usually can provide the most comprehensive and accurate ADL information. Discussions with family members, documentation in the medical record, and observation of the resident can also help staff members accurately code this item.

Code bed mobility, transferring, eating, and toileting according to the resident's actual self-performance, not what is anticipated or expected. Bed mobility includes the resident's ability to move and reposition while in bed, turn from side to side, and move to and from a lying position. Transferring excludes transfers to and from the toilet or bath but does include all transfers between bed, chair (wheelchair or stationary), or a standing position. Eating excludes setting up a tray or plate but includes actual intake via any route (oral, intravenous, or tube feedings). Toilet use assesses transfers to and from the toilet or commode and self-performance when using the toileting facilities, including cleansing and adjusting clothing.

ADL support provided

When determining the amount of assistance required for bed mobility, transferring, eating, and toileting, carefully read and study the description of each level of assistance. Staff must understand and appropriately code the amount and frequency of oversight, encouragement, physical assistance, non–weight-bearing support, and weight-bearing support.

Follow all of the preceding rules and guidelines when coding the remaining ADL items in section G1 (non–late-loss ADLs). These six ADLs are walking in the room (G1c), walking in the corridor (G1d), locomotion on the unit (G1e), locomotion off the unit (G1f), dressing (G1g), and personal hygiene (G1j). If you code a resident as totally dependent, meaning that the resident performed none of the preceding activities, this resident would not be considered for the quality indicator. Coding item B1 as a 1 (having a diagnosis of coma or persistent vegetative state) would also exclude the resident.

Proper assessment in this area of the ADL status is important for a correct reflection of any decline or improvement. MDS assessors should carefully examine the ADL status when they determine that a decline occurred. Because two MDS forms are being compared, if two different assessors completed the forms, the reliability and continuity of the assessment become important. All personnel completing this portion of the MDS should ensure proper coding that reflects actual resident status as described by the definitions of each numerical code.

Regulatory agencies will examine a nursing facility with a high percentage of residents with a decline in ADLs to determine whether this decline was preventable. If the nursing home had a high number of critically ill, unstable residents, this decline in ADLs may be expected. However, if the decline was preventable (i.e., through increased staffing or improved care planning), the lack of quality of care requires further investigation.

Quality indicator 18: Incidence of decline in range of motion

Basic information

- **Indicator type:** Quality indicator 18, the final indicator in the physical functioning domain, is also an incidence indicator. Data from two MDS forms are used for the potential flagging of this indicator: the current MDS (excluding the initial admission assessment) and the prior MDS assessment. A comparison of these two assessments will show whether there has been a change in ROM status over time.
- **Facility percentage:** Surveyors analyze the facility percentage, which is calculated by comparing those residents who had an increase in ROM functional limitation over two MDS assessments with all residents who have two completed MDS assessments. Residents who already have the maximum amount of numerically coded functional limitations, and therefore cannot decline any further, are excluded from the denominator of the facility percentage.
- **Risk adjustment:** Quality indicator 18 is not risk adjusted.

Related MDS items

Section G—physical functioning and structural problems—again provides the data for quality indicator 18. Specifically, functional limitation in ROM (G4a–f box A) is assessed. Box B, voluntary movement, does not contribute to the determination of the flagging of this indicator.

Six areas are assessed for ROM in this section of the MDS: neck, arm, hand, leg, foot, and any other limitation. Staff should use a seven-day assessment period, ending on the MDS assessment reference date. Score each of these six areas using one of three numerical codes depending on the amount of limitation present with ROM. A score of 0 means no limitation, 1 means limitation only on one side of the body, and 2 means limitation on both sides of the body.

After you code items G4a–f box A according to the preceding description, the numerical codes in these six boxes are added together. If the sum of the six boxes is greater on the current assessment than on the prior assessment, a decline in ROM has occurred, and this indicator is present. If the sum of the boxes on the current assessment is the same or less than the sum of the prior assessment, the indicator is not present. This comparison shows either an improvement or no change in ROM status.

If you code a score of 2 in each item G4a–f box A, the sum of 12 for all six areas is the maximum amount of ROM limitation. Therefore, ROM could not decline any further, and a resident with this coding in the previous MDS assessment is excluded from the determination of the facility percentage.

MDS assessment and coding

Range of motion

Staff should assess ROM according to limitations present only during the seven-day assessment period ending with the assessment reference date of the MDS. You should not code limitations that were present but resolved before this assessment period. Coding for ROM limitations depends on the extent of each limitation and where the limitation presents itself.

Assessors should test each of the six areas in items G4a–f box A with actual ROM exercises to accurately code for these items (Figure 10.1). If the resident is cognitively capable of performing the ROM test for each area identified, the assessor observes for limitations, questions the resident about their perception of any difficulties, and completes the assessment. For those residents unable to perform the tests independently, the MDS assessor should perform active assisted ROM. This test should be done very gently and stopped immediately if the resident indicates any type of pain. The presence of a fracture or surgical site would negate the need to perform the test for that area.

Figure 10.1

Testing the Range of Motion

Specific tests for ROM limitations are identified and explained in the *RAI User's Manual*. A brief summary of each test is listed below:

- **Neck:** Resident turns head side to side and shoulder to shoulder.
- **Arm:** Resident lifts arms to place hands behind head and touch each shoulder with opposite hand.
- **Hand:** Resident makes a fist and opens hand.
- **Leg:** While lying flat, resident lifts each leg bending it at the knee.
- **Foot:** Resident flexes and extends each foot.
- **Other:** Resident has a limitation in joints not listed above.

After performing the tests in Figure 10.1, the assessor can determine whether no limitations are present, a ROM limitation exists on one side of the body, or the limitation is present on both sides of the body. A unilateral amputation is coded a 1 (limitation on one side) whereas a bilateral amputation is coded a 2 (limitation on both sides).

Regulatory agencies will investigate a nursing center with a high percentage of residents who had a decline in ROM to determine the reason for this decline. Scrutinize the restorative program to determine its effectiveness, and conduct an evaluation of the therapy department's involvement. If the decline in ROM could have been prevented, quality of care could be in question.

At a Glance

Domain #8
Physical Functioning

Quality Indicators	MDS Items	MDS Codes
16. Prevalence of bedfast residents	G6a: Bedfast all or most of time	Box is checked
17. Incidence of decline in late-loss ADLs	G1a Box A: Bed mobility self-performance	0 on previous MDS and 1, 2, 3, or 4 on current MDS
		1 on previous MDS and 2, 3, or 4 on current MDS
		2 on previous MDS and 3 or 4 on current MDS
		3 on previous MDS and 4 on current MDS
	G1b Box A: Transfer self-performance	0 on previous MDS and 1, 2, 3, or 4 on current MDS
		1 on previous MDS and 2, 3, or 4 on current MDS

Domain #8 (cont.)

Quality Indicators	MDS Items	MDS Codes
See previous page.	See previous page.	2 on previous MDS and 3 or 4 on current MDS
		3 on previous MDS and 4 on current MDS
	G1h Box A: Eating self-performance	0 on previous MDS and 1, 2, 3, or 4 on current MDS
		1 on previous MDS and 2, 3, or 4 on current MDS
		2 on previous MDS and 3 or 4 on current MDS
		3 on previous MDS and 4 on current MDS
	G1i Box A: Toilet use self-performance	0 on previous MDS and 1, 2, 3, or 4 on current MDS
		1 on previous MDS and 2, 3, or 4 on current MDS

Domain #8 (cont.)

Quality Indicators	MDS Items	MDS Codes
See previous page.	See previous page.	2 on previous MDS and 3 or 4 on current MDS
		3 on previous MDS and 4 on current MDS
	Two ADLs changed from above or one from below:	
	G1a Box A: Bed mobility self-performance	0 on previous MDS and 2, 3, or 4 on current MDS
		1 on previous MDS and 3 or 4 on current MDS
		2 on previous MDS and 4 on current MDS
	G1b Box A: Transfer self-performance	0 on previous MDS and 2, 3, or 4 on current MDS
		1 on previous MDS and 3 or 4 on current MDS

Domain #8 (cont.)

Quality Indicators	MDS Items	MDS Codes
See previous page.	See previous page.	2 on previous MDS and 4 on current MDS
	G1h Box A: Eating self-performance	0 on previous MDS and 2, 3, or 4 on current MDS
		1 on previous MDS and 3 or 4 on current MDS
		2 on previous MDS and 4 on current MDS
	G1i Box A: Toilet use self-performance	0 on previous MDS and 2, 3, or 4 on current MDS
		1 on previous MDS and 3 or 4 on current MDS
		2 on previous MDS and 4 on current MDS
Exclusion of residents for QI #17	B1: Comatose	1
	OR	
	G1a Box A: Bed mobility self-performance	4 or 8

Domain #8 (cont.)

Quality Indicators	MDS Items	MDS Codes
See previous page.	G1b Box A: Transfer self-performance	4 or 8, and;
	G1c Box A: Walk in room self-performance	4 or 8, and;
	G1d Box A: Walk in corridor self-performance	4 or 8, and;
	G1e Box A: Locomotion on unit self-performance	4 or 8, and;
	G1f Box A: Locomotion off unit self-performance	4 or 8, and;
	G1g Box A: Dressing self-performance	4 or 8, and;
	G1h Box A: Eating self-performance	4 or 8, and;
	G1i Box A: Toilet use self-performance	4 or 8, and;
	G1j Box A: Personal hygiene self-performance	4 or 8

Domain #8 (cont.)

Quality Indicators	MDS Items	MDS Codes
18. Incidence of decline in ROM	G4a Box A: Neck ROM G4b Box A: Arm ROM G4c Box A: Hand ROM G4d Box A: Leg ROM G4e Box A: Foot ROM G4f Box A: Other ROM	Sum total of values 0, 1, and 2 in six areas of ROM is greater on current MDS than on previous MDS
Exclusion of residents for QI #18	G4a Box A: Neck ROM	2 and;
	G4b Box A: Arm ROM	2 and;
	G4c Box A: Hand ROM	2 and;
	G4d Box A: Leg ROM	2 and;
	G4e Box A: Foot ROM	2 and;
	G4f Box A: Other ROM	2 on previous MDS

Chapter 11

Psychotropic Drug Use Domain

The major emphasis of the psychotropic drug use domain is similar to the clinical management domain. Both domains deal with medication use, but this area specifically addresses the use of psychotropic drugs.

The presence of cognitive impairment and psychological conditions in the elderly nursing home population makes the correct and proper use of these medications critical. Overuse can result in numerous adverse side effects, including excessive lethargy, decreased appetite, and potential for injury from falling. Underuse can lead to uncontrolled and distressing behavior problems. The following three quality indicators are included in this domain:

- Prevalence of antipsychotic use in the absence of psychotic and related conditions
- Prevalence of antianxiety/hypnotic medication use
- Prevalence of hypnotic medication use more than two times in last week

Proper use of all psychotropic drugs can help control behaviors and enhance a resident's quality of life.

Quality indicator 19: Prevalence of antipsychotic use in the absence of psychotic or related conditions

Basic information

- **Indicator type:** Quality indicator 19, the first indicator in the psychotropic drug use domain, is a prevalence indicator and uses data from the most recently completed MDS assessment (excluding the initial admission assessment).

- **Facility percentage:** Surveyors analyze the facility percentage, which is derived by comparing all residents who received antipsychotic medication as coded on the MDS assessment with all residents in the facility who have a completed MDS, excluding those residents who have a psychotic or related disorder.

- **Risk adjustment:** Quality indicator 19 is risk adjusted depending on the presence of cognitive impairment and behavioral problems.

Related MDS items

The MDS item antipsychotic medications (O4a) provides the primary data for this indicator. Staff should code this item according to the number of days the resident received antipsychotic medication within the seven-day assessment period ending with the MDS assessment reference date. Coding for this item ranges from 0 (an antipsychotic was not used) to 7 (an antipsychotic was administered every day during the previous seven-day period). Score antipsychotics that are long-acting and administered less than weekly as a 1 in item O4a.

If a resident receives an antipsychotic medication and has a psychotic diagnosis, you should exclude him or her from the facility percentage. Section I, disease diagnoses, and item J1i, hallucinations, contain the information to obtain this exclusion. If you check any one of the following items, or if you enter a specific diagnosis in other current or more detailed diagnoses and ICD-9 codes (I3), a psychotic or related condition is present:

- Schizophrenia (I1gg) is checked
- Hallucinations (J1i) is checked
- I3 has an ICD-9 code of 307.23: Tourette's disorder
- I3 has an ICD-9 code of 333.4: Huntington's chorea
- I3 has an ICD-9 code of 295.00–295.9: Schizophrenic disorders
- I3 has an ICD-9 code of 297.00–298.9: Paranoid or delusional disorders or other nonorganic psychoses

Only one of the preceding conditions or diagnoses must be present for a resident to have what is defined as a psychotic or related condition. Once again, if the most recent MDS was a quarterly assessment, you can obtain the preceding information from the most recent full assessment. With the exception of hallucinations, the quarterly does not include this diagnosis information.

Weighing the risk factor

The risk adjustment of quality indicator 19 results in more MDS items to consider. The presence of the combination of cognitive impairment and behavior problems places a resident in the high-risk category for antipsychotic use with no psychotic or related conditions. Staff will need to code all of the following MDS items as follows for both cognitive impairment and behavior problems to be present:

- B4 is scored a 1, 2, or 3
- B2a is scored a 1
- E4b, E4c, or E4d box A is scored a 1, 2, or 3

These MDS items—cognitive impairment and behavior problems—are also important for quality indicators discussed previously. The quality indicator 3 risk adjustment—prevalence of behavioral symptoms affecting others—and quality indicator 7—incidence of cognitive impairment—both deal with this same cognitive impairment. Behavioral symptoms on the MDS also influence quality indicator 3.

To review, you should code item B4 (cognitive skills for daily decision making) depending on the amount of impairment present with decision-making processes during the previous seven-day assessment period. A 0 means independence with daily decisions, 1 means modified independence, 2 means moderate impairment, and 3 means severe impairment.

Item B2a addresses a resident's short-term memory. If a resident has good short-term recall, code this item a 0. The inability to recall concepts or events after five minutes results in a score of 1. You should assess this item using the usual 7-day assessment period.

Staff should assess Section E4, behavioral symptoms, according to the frequency of behaviors present during the previous seven days. For quality indicator 19, as with quality indicator 3, staff should assess only the frequency of the behaviors, not their alterability. Code verbally abusive, physically abusive, and socially inappropriate or disruptive behaviors according to the number of days that those specific behaviors occurred. If the behavior was not present, the score is 0; if the behavior was present 1–3 days, the score is 1; if the behavior is present 4–6 days, the score is 2; and if the behavior is present every day, the score is 3.

If assessors do not code both cognitive impairment and behavior problems according to the preceding MDS item definitions, the resident is considered to be at low risk. The presence of only one of the preceding two conditions also results in a low-risk placement. No further MDS items are used for the categorization of low risk.

MDS assessment and coding

Item O4a, antipsychotic, is the primary MDS item that affects the flagging of quality indicator 19. It is therefore extremely important to code this item correctly. To accurately determine whether a medication is in the antipsychotic class of drugs, staff can use a reference manual such as the *PDR*. Further, new medications are always being introduced, so consultation with a pharmacist can also assist staff in coding this item correctly.

Antipsychotic use

When assessing for antipsychotic use, code only the number of days that the antipsychotic was actually administered, not just that it was ordered by the physician. For example, if a resident refuses the medication for a day, or if the medication was held for a day because of a pending diagnostic test, do not include that day when coding this item.

Staff should assess antipsychotic medication administered by any route, including the oral, intramuscular, intravenous, and enteral routes. Staff should also use the seven-day assessment time frame, even if the resident was not at the nursing center the entire time. If the resident was sent to an emergency room or outpatient clinic and an antipsychotic medication was administered there, include that day in the final code for this item. Additionally, if a resident new to the nursing center received antipsychotic medication before transfer to the nursing facility, and the period is within the seven-day assessment time frame, also count these days.

Staff can verify the number of days antipsychotic drugs are given during the assessment period by looking at the medication administration record. Count these days and code accordingly in item O4a. If the resident received a long-acting antipsychotic drug, but not within the seven-day period, code a score of 1. A score of 1 or higher could cause the indicator to flag depending on the resident's current diagnosis.

Exclusion of residents

A diagnosis of schizophrenia (I1gg) excludes the resident from the facility percentage for quality indicator 19 and should be checked if applicable. Staff can confirm a diagnosis of schizophrenia by consulting medical record documentation. As mentioned previously, specific diagnoses entered in other current or more detailed diagnoses and ICD-9 codes (I3) that exclude a resident from this indicator are Tourette's disorder, Huntington's chorea, and other psychotic disorders such as paranoid states and nonorganic psychoses. When considering diagnoses and codes in item I3, enter any active current diagnoses that affect the resident's health or behavioral status. Either consulting with the physician or reviewing the medical record documentation can assist in determining these diagnoses.

Hallucinations (J1i) is the final condition that excludes a resident from the facility percentage. Hallucinations are defined in the revised *RAI User's Manual* as false perceptions occurring without actual, true stimuli. These perceptions can be visual, auditory, tactile, olfactory, or gustatory in nature. Staff can assess the presence of hallucinations within the previous seven-day period by directly questioning the resident about whether any of the preceding perceptions occurred and by reviewing the documentation in the medical record. Staff and family members can also provide information for this assessment.

Assessing for cognitive impairment and behavioral symptoms was addressed in the discussion of quality indicators 3 and 7. To briefly review, staff can assess daily decision making by monitoring the resident's decision-making abilities in his or her current environment. Staff should directly observe and question the resident or discuss the issue with other staff members and the resident's family. Asking the resident to remember a set of items or ideas and then questioning the resident whether he or she can recall the information can be a good way to assess for short-term memory problems. Assess both decision making and short-term memory using the seven-day period ending with the MDS assessment reference date.

Assessors can either directly observe the behaviors of verbal abuse, physical abuse, or socially inappropriate/disruptive actions or review the documentation in the medical record. Once again, assessors should consult with all staff members on all shifts to determine whether these behaviors were present at any time. You should use the usual seven-day assessment period.

If a nursing home has a high percentage of residents receiving antipsychotic medications without a psychotic diagnosis, investigation is warranted to determine why these residents are receiving the medication. A facility's specialization in the care of cognitively impaired or other psychologically impaired residents may explain the high percentage. On the other hand, antipsychotics used solely for behavior control because of the staff's unwillingness to deal with these behaviors would warrant further investigation of quality of care issues.

Quality indicator 20: Prevalence of antianxiety/hypnotic use

Basic information

- **Indicator type:** Quality indicator 20 is the second quality indicator in the psychotropic drug use domain and is a prevalence indicator. Only data from the most recently completed MDS is considered (excluding the initial admission assessment).

- **Facility percentage:** Surveyors analyze the facility percentage, which is arrived at by comparing all residents who received antianxiety or hypnotic medication with all residents who have a completed MDS assessment. The identical exclusions discussed with quality indicator 19 are also present with indicator 20: Residents with psychotic or related conditions are not included.

- **Risk adjustment:** Quality indicator 20 is not risk adjusted.

Related MDS items

Two MDS items are of primary importance for this indicator. Section O, medications, provides this information, specifically the MDS items antianxiety (O4b) and hypnotic (O4d). As in the previous indicator for antipsychotic medications, you should code these two items depending on the number of days a resident received either an antianxiety or hypnotic medication. A range of 0 to 7 is possible, 0 designating no use of the medication and 7 referring to daily administration. You should code a long-acting medication used less than weekly as a 1. Use the usual seven-day assessment period ending with the MDS assessment reference date.

Exclusion of residents

The identical diagnoses and presence of hallucinations of quality indicator 19 exclude residents from the facility percentage for indicator 20. The diagnoses and coding are as follows:

- Schizophrenia (I1gg) is checked
- Hallucinations (J1i) is checked
- I3 has an ICD-9 code of 307.23: Tourette's disorder
- I3 has an ICD-9 code of 333.4: Huntington's chorea
- I3 has an ICD-9 code of 295.00–295.9: Schizophrenic disorders
- I3 has an ICD-9 code of 297.00–298.9: Paranoid/delusional disorders or other nonorganic psychoses

As with quality indicator 19, only one of the preceding conditions excludes the resident from the indicator 20 calculation because of the resulting need for the antianxiety or hypnotic medication. If the most recently completed MDS is a quarterly assessment, the most recent full MDS assessment is used to derive this information about diseases. With the exception of hallucinations, this information is not on the quarterly form.

MDS assessment and coding

Assessors should code both antianxiety medication (O4b) and hypnotic medication (O4d) using the same method as in quality indicator 19, which considers antipsychotic medication. Only antianxiety or hypnotic medication coded as received during the previous seven days flags quality indicator 20. Both drug classes do not need to be present for the potential flagging to occur.

The antianxiety or hypnotic medication can be received by any route, including oral, intravenous, intramuscular, or enteral. Consider any setting, in addition to the nursing facility, in which the resident received the medication, including hospitals, outpatient clinics, or doctors' offices. Staff can use the nursing home administration record or records from other healthcare facilities to determine the accurate codes for these items during the assessment period.

Once again, it is important to accurately classify these medications. Antianxiety and hypnotic medications can have similar pharmacologic properties; therefore, consulting a pharmacist or using a reference book such as the *PDR* is advisable. In the final coding of these items, only include medications that were actually administered.

Assessors complete coding of diseases by reviewing the diagnoses listed in the resident's medical chart or by discussing this information with the physician. As explained in the quality indicator 19 discussion, they should enter only those active diagnoses pertaining to the resident's current health and behavioral status in other current or more detailed diagnoses and ICD-9 codes (I3). Any of the specific preceding diagnoses listed exclude the resident from consideration for the facility percentage. The presence of hallucinations as evidenced by resident and staff reports or chart documentation is the final exclusion.

If many residents without psychotic conditions are receiving either antianxiety or hypnotic medications, this raises a question about whether there was a need for these medications. Substantiating conditions and proper nursing care could cause surveyors to conclude that quality of care is present. Inability to explain why residents are receiving these medications would result in further scrutiny by regulatory agencies.

Quality indicator 21: Prevalence of hypnotic use more than two times in the last week

Basic information

- **Indicator type:** Quality indicator 21, the final indicator in the psychotropic drug use domain, is also a prevalence indicator. Data from only the most recently completed MDS assessment are included (excluding the initial admission assessment).

- **Facility percentage:** Surveyors analyze the facility percentage, which is determined by comparing those residents who received hypnotic medication on more than two days in the previous seven-day period with all residents who have a completed MDS assessment. Unlike the other two quality indicators in this domain, no denominator exclusion is used.

- **Risk adjustment:** Quality indicator 21 is not risk adjusted.

Related MDS item

Only one MDS item provides data for quality indicator 21—hypnotic medication (O4d). Assessors should code the item depending on the number of days within the seven-day assessment period that a hypnotic medication was administered; therefore, the coding ranges from 0 (no hypnotic used) to 7 (hypnotic used on a daily basis). As explained previously, always code a long-acting hypnotic administered less than weekly as a 1. If you assign this item a code greater than a 2—that is, a score of 3 through 7—the indicator will flag.

Assessment and coding

Because the coding of O4d directly affects the flagging of two quality indicators (numbers 20 and 21), it is extremely important that assessors score this item accurately. No residents are excluded from the potential flagging; every resident receiving a hypnotic medication more than twice a week is reflected in the facility percentage. Therefore, it is vital that staff code medications correctly in section O4 and that they accurately identify hypnotics. The importance of consulting the *PDR* cannot be overemphasized. For example, an assessor might code a drug as a hypnotic when in fact the correct classification is an antidepressant or antianxiety medication.

Assessors must consider all hypnotics administered using any route (e.g., oral, parenteral, intravenous, or intramuscular) and in any setting (nursing home, physician's office, hospital, or clinic). Include only medications actually given to the resident, not those simply ordered. For example, you should not count a hypnotic ordered prn in the evening, but not actually administered. If a resident refuses the medication, do not include it in the scoring of this item.

When assessing this item, use the typical seven-day time period, ending with the MDS assessment reference date. The assessor must accurately determine the seven-day period to count the correct number of days the medication was administered. For example, an assessment reference date on a Thursday only looks back to the previous Friday, not the previous Thursday. Review medication administration records for the number of days hypnotics were administered in order to code this item.

Regulatory agencies will inspect a nursing facility with a high rate of hypnotic use to determine why these medications were administered. Using hypnotic medications to promote sleep in patients without a valid reason for doing so raises questions about whether the medication is being used solely for staff convenience. A definite and documented reason and physical condition for the use could indicate an awareness of quality of care.

At a Glance

Domain #9
Psychotropic Drug Use

Quality Indicators	MDS Items	MDS Codes
19. Prevalence of antipsychotic use, in the absence of psychotic and related conditions	O4a: Antipsychotics	1, 2, 3, 4, 5, 6, or 7
Exclusion of residents for QI #19	I1gg: Schizophrenia	Box is checked, or;
	J1i: Hallucinations	Box is checked, or;
	I3: Other current or more detailed diagnoses and ICD-9 codes	Diagnosis ICD-9 code is 295.00–295.9, 297.00–298.9, 307.23, or 333.4
High risk for QI #19	B4: Cognitive skills for daily decision-making	1, 2, or 3, and;
	B2a: Short-term memory	1
	AND	

Domain #9 (cont.)

Quality Indicators	MDS Items	MDS Codes
See previous page.	E4b Box A: Verbally abusive behavioral symptoms frequency	1, 2, or 3, or;
	E4c Box A: Physically abusive behavioral symptoms frequency	1, 2, or 3, or;
	E4d Box A: Socially inappropriate/disruptive behavioral symptoms frequency	1, 2, or 3
Low risk for QI #19—all other residents not classified as high risk	N/A	N/A
20. Prevalence of antianxiety/hypnotic use	O4b: Antianxiety	1, 2, 3, 4, 5, 6, or 7, or;
	O4d: Hypnotic	1, 2, 3, 4, 5, 6, or 7
Exclusion of residents for QI #20	I1gg: Schizophrenia	Box is checked, or;
	J1i: Hallucinations	Box is checked, or;
	I3: Other current or more detailed diagnoses and ICD-9 codes	Diagnosis ICD-9 code is 295.00–295.9, 297.00–298.9, 307.23, or 333.4

Domain #9 (cont.)

Quality Indicators	MDS Items	MDS Codes
21. Prevalence of hypnotic use more than two times in last week	O4d: Hypnotic	3, 4, 5, 6, or 7

Chapter 12

Quality of Life Domain

A resident's quality of life in a nursing center encompasses many different areas of daily living. Alleviation of pain, contact with family and friends, and being able to pursue a desired daily lifestyle are just a few of these areas. A nursing center that assists with and promotes the resident's ability to lead his or her life as wished is attempting to maintain this quality at the highest level possible. Although CHSRA states that the other domains include quality of life indicators, two specific areas are considered for this domain: prevalence of daily physical restraints and prevalence of little or no activity. A low number of residents with either of these scenarios shows an increased potential for high quality of life.

Quality indicator 22: Prevalence of daily physical restraints

Basic information

- **Indicator type:** The data obtained for quality indicator 22, the first indicator in the quality of life domain, comes from the most recently completed MDS assessment (excluding the initial admission assessment).

- **Facility percentage:** Surveyors analyze the facility percentage, which is determined by comparing those residents who were physically restrained on a daily basis with all other residents who have a completed MDS assessment.

- **Risk adjustment:** Quality indicator 22 is not risk adjusted.

Related MDS items

Three MDS items provide information for quality indicator 22. In section P—special treatments and procedures—trunk restraints (P4c), limb restraints (P4d), and chairs that prevent rising (P4e) provide data about physical restraints. For quality indicator 22, bed rails are not classified as physical restraints.

Staff can assess the use of each of the three preceding types of restraints by considering the usual seven-day assessment period, ending with the MDS assessment reference date. Possible codes for these restraints are 0, the restraints were not used during the assessment period; 1, the restraints were used less than daily (1–6 days); or 2, the restraints were used daily. If you code any one of P4c, P4d, or P4e a 2, this quality indicator will flag. Only one daily restraint is required for flagging; all three do not need to be used.

MDS assessment and coding

To accurately code items P4c, P4d, and P4e, consider the exact definition of each restraint. Restraints are devices that restrict movement and cannot be easily removed by the resident. Any devices that the resident can easily remove, such as a self-releasing wheelchair belt, are not considered restraints.

Trunk restraints are applied to the upper or central part of the body and include waist or vest restraints. Limb restraints are applied to a limb or any part of a limb and include restraints for both the arms and legs. Wrist or ankle restraints are examples of limb restraints. Chairs that prevent rising are defined as any type of chair that does not allow the resident to rise easily. This includes geri-chairs with locked lap boards, reclining geri-chairs restricting rising, merry walkers, and the application of lap buddies.

Staff can assess restraint use by directly observing the resident and by consulting documentation in the medical record. Questioning staff members on all shifts also helps determine whether restraints were used at any time during the seven-day assessment period.

Regulatory agencies will investigate a nursing center with a high percentage of residents with restraints to determine whether the restraints are used appropriately and whether methods are currently in place for restraint reduction. The level of staffing at the facility could also be checked to discover whether the restraints are used more for staff ease and convenience than for resident need. All of the preceding considerations should be investigated to determine whether quality of life is present.

Quality indicator 23: Prevalence of little or no activity

Basic information

- Indicator type: Quality indicator 23 is a prevalence indicator that obtains data from the most recently completed MDS assessment (excluding the initial admission assessment).

- **Facility percentage:** Surveyors analyze the facility percentage, which is determined by comparing those residents coded as having little or no activity with all residents who have a completed MDS assessment, with one exclusion: Residents who are comatose and therefore unable to participate in activities are not included.

- **Risk adjustment:** Quality indicator 23 is not risk adjusted.

Related MDS items

Activity pursuit patterns are addressed on the MDS in section N. Item N2 assesses the average time involved in daily activities and should be coded according to the previous seven-day assessment period, ending with the MDS assessment reference date. You can enter one of four possible codes in item N2: A score of 0 means that the resident is involved in activities more than two-thirds of the time; 1 means the resident is involved one-third to two-thirds of the time; 2 means the resident is involved less than one-third of the time; and 3 means no involvement in activities. The available time assessed for participating in activities excludes time spent sleeping and receiving treatments or daily cares.

Average time involved in daily activities

If you code item N2 as a 2 (little activity involvement) or a 3 (no activities), this quality indicator will flag unless you coded item B1 as a 1, meaning the resident is in a coma or a persistent vegetative state. The presence of a coma and little or no activities will not affect the facility percentage for this quality indicator.

MDS assessment and coding

What counts as an activity?

Proper coding of the amount of time a resident is involved in activities is crucial. Staff must also understand the definition of what constitutes an activity. Activities can include those structured, planned events coordinated by the activity department of the nursing facility, such as bingo, holiday parties, and group outings. Many assessors, however, do not include solitary activities in their assessments. Watching birds outside a window, sitting in the hallway interacting with other residents and staff, reading a book or magazine, or talking with a roommate are all examples of activities that you should include in the total time involved in activities coded in item N2.

As mentioned previously, the total amount of time a resident is considered capable of participating in activities should not include time spent receiving ADL care, therapy treatments, or medications. Additionally, exclude time spent sleeping from the total available time.

Gathering the data

When assessing activity, question the resident directly to determine activity involvement. Even if he or she is not participating in structured activities, a resident might still be involved in solitary activities of his or her choosing. Direct caregivers who observe the resident on a routine basis can also provide assessment information; assessors should also review medical chart documentation when completing this MDS item.

Where do you stand?

Regulatory agencies will investigate a nursing home with a high percentage of residents participating in little or no activity to determine whether there is a lack of available activities, residents are not encouraged to participate in activities, or residents choose not to become involved. Undercoding of this item could also result in an artificially high percentage of residents appearing uninvolved. Further scrutiny will assist in determining whether a quality of life issue exists.

At a Glance

Domain #10
Quality of Life

Quality Indicators	MDS Items	MDS Codes
22. Prevalence of daily physical restraints	P4c: Trunk restraint	2, or;
	P4d: Limb restraint	2, or;
	P4e: Chair prevents rising	2
23. Prevalence of little or no activity	N2: Average time involved in activities	2 or 3
Exclusion of residents for QI #23	B1: Comatose	1

Chapter 13

Skin Care Domain

The maintenance of healthy skin relates to many areas of a resident's overall care status. Adequate nourishment and hydration, frequent repositioning, and incontinence management all play a major role in good skin care and have been identified as quality indicators in previous domains. Only one quality indicator, prevalence of stage 1–4 pressure ulcers, is included in this domain. The prevalence of pressure ulcers in low-risk residents, which is part of this quality indicator, is the third designated sentinel event.

Quality indicator 24: Prevalence of stage 1–4 pressure ulcers

Basic information

- **Indicator type:** Quality indicator 24, the final quality indicator, is a prevalence indicator, and data for the facility percentage are obtained from the most recently completed MDS assessment (excluding the initial admission assessment).
- **Facility percentage:** Surveyors analyze the facility percentage, which is calculated by comparing all residents who have a stage 1–4 pressure ulcer with all residents in the facility who have a completed MDS assessment.

- **Risk adjustment:** Quality indicator 24 is divided into high-risk and low-risk categories depending on the ADL status and presence of specific diagnoses. Any situation in which a low-risk resident develops pressure ulcers qualifies as a sentinel event. Regulatory agencies consider even one resident in this category serious enough to require intensive review and investigation to determine the reason for the occurrence.

Related MDS items

Section M—skin condition—provides the majority of information for quality indicator 24. Staff should code the first item, ulcers (M1), according to the number of ulcers and open lesions and which stage each appears at on the resident's body. If no ulcer is present at a specified stage, you should code the stage a 0. If ulcers are present, enter the number of ulcers in the box for that stage. If nine or more ulcers exist at a certain stage, the code is 9.

The item pressure ulcers (M2a) directly contributes to the potential flagging of this indicator. Code M2a according to the highest stage of pressure ulcers identified in item M1. The range of values for this item is 0 (no pressure ulcers) to 4 (a stage 4 pressure ulcer coded in item M1). A code of stage 1, 2, 3, or 4 in item M2a designating the presence of a pressure ulcer in M1 causes quality indicator 24 to be present. The coding of a stasis ulcer (M2b) does not affect the indicator.

Both items M1 and M2a assess the skin condition during the previous seven-day assessment period. The seven-day time frame ends with the MDS assessment reference date and only includes pressure ulcers present during that period. Ulcers before the assessment period are not coded.

What causes the indicator to flag?

Even if you code item M2a as a 0 (no pressure ulcer present), indicator 24 may flag if other current or more detailed diagnoses and ICD-9 codes (I3) is 707.0, the code for decubitus ulcers. Item I3 only includes current and active diagnoses affecting the resident's health and behavioral status. If a resident has this decubitus ulcer diagnosis, it is entered in item I3.

Assessing risk

The risk adjustment for quality indicator 24 results in more MDS items to consider. If a resident has ADL dependence needs or specific conditions and diagnoses, the resident could be placed in the high-risk category. The coding of either bed mobility (G1a) or transferring (G1b) in the physical functioning and structural problems section of the MDS affects the risk adjustment. As in the risk adjustment for quality indicator 8 (prevalence of bladder or bowel incontinence) and quality indicator 17 (incidence of decline in late loss ADLs), only the coding in the self-performance column is considered. If you code bed mobility or transferring self-performance as a 3 (extensive assistance) or a 4 (total dependence), the resident is placed in the high-risk category for pressure ulcer development because of the potential for immobility.

High-risk residents

Various other conditions and diagnoses also impact the risk adjustment for indicator 24. If you code any one of the following MDS items as listed, the resident is considered to be high risk:

- B1 (comatose) is scored a 1
- J5c (end-stage disease) is checked

- I3 has an ICD-9 code of 260, 261, 262, 263.0, 263.1, 263.2, 263.8, or 263.9

Only one of the preceding diagnoses or conditions must be present to result in the high-risk status.

Low-risk residents

If a resident has neither bed mobility or transferring dependence, nor one of the preceding conditions or diagnoses, the resident is at low risk for pressure ulcer development. As discussed earlier in this chapter, if a resident develops a pressure ulcer and is at low risk for that development, a sentinel event has occurred, necessitating intense scrutiny of possible regulatory and quality-of-care issues.

MDS assessment and coding

Ulcers

To determine quality of care, or lack thereof, in the skin care domain, it is critical to code M1 of the MDS accurately (Figure 13.1). Miscoding of this item can result in an artificially high percentage of residents flagging quality indicator 24 or the incorrect presence of a sentinel event.

The most appropriate and comprehensive clinical method for determining the presence of any of the four stages of ulcers listed in Figure 13.1 is to perform a complete skin examination of the resident. Bony prominences should be studied extremely carefully to note any redness or open areas. Reviewing the medical chart and questioning nursing staff members will assist with this assessment. Staff should then record the presence of any ulcers and use the appropriate codes on the MDS.

Figure 13.1

Identifying the Correct Stage

On the MDS form, each of the four stages of ulcers is identified and defined:

- **Stage 1:** Persistent area of redness with no break in the skin, that does not go away when pressure is relieved.
- **Stage 2:** Partial loss of skin layers to include a blister, abrasion, or shallow open area.
- **Stage 3:** Full loss of skin layers exposing the subcutaneous tissues exhibited as a deep open area.
- **Stage 4:** Full loss of skin and subcutaneous tissues; muscle and/or bone is exposed.

Using a seven-day assessment period, enter the stage of any ulcer during that time period in item M1. The MDS completion directions state that if necrotic eschar is present, the ulcer is always coded a stage 4 until the eschar is débrided and accurate staging can occur. Additionally, ulcers resulting from circulatory issues, pressure or diseases such as syphillis are considered for item M1. Pressure and poor circulation are two common reasons ulcers develop, which are then differentiated in item M2.

Certain skin conditions should not be coded in item M1, ulcers, but rather in item M4, other skin problems or lesions present. These include rashes without a break in the skin, burns, desensitized skin, and surgical openings.

Coding of item M2a directly determines a resident's potential inclusion in the facility percentage for possible flagging. The presence of pressure ulcers only, not stasis ulcers, affects quality indicator 24. Therefore, it is necessary to have a clear understanding of the definition of both types of ulcers.

Pressure ulcers

As the name implies, a pressure ulcer is caused by pressure placed on a part of the body for a length of time, resulting in damaged skin tissues. Redness that does not disappear easily is usually the first sign of a pressure ulcer. Continued pressure, especially on a bony prominence, can result in an open area on the skin that can progress down to muscle or bone, or both.

Stasis ulcers

Stasis ulcers, as defined in the MDS manual, are caused by a decrease in blood flow due to venous insufficiency. These ulcers are not a result of increased prolonged pressure to an area of the skin and are not considered for quality indicator 24. Reviewing diagnoses (e.g., peripheral vascular disease), questioning staff members, and/or consulting with the physician can assist in determining whether ulcers are stasis ulcers.

When coding M2, you must classify the ulcers identified in M1 properly according to their cause. Code in M2a only the ulcers clearly identified as caused by pressure. Do not consider ulcers resulting from other causes for this item. When coding M2a, you should enter only the highest-stage pressure ulcer. For example, if a resident has a stage 3 stasis ulcer and a stage 2 pressure ulcer, score item M2a as a 2, not a 3.

Other current or more detailed diagnoses

Other current or more detailed diagnoses and ICD-9 codes (I3) is the second area of the MDS to provide data for indicator 24. Item I3 includes those current active diagnoses that affect the resident's physical health and behavioral status. The presence of the decubitus ulcer code, 707.0, even if M2a does not indicate an ulcer, will flag indicator 24. If a resident has this diagnosis due to a decubitus ulcer in the distant past that is now healed, and no further ulcer development has occurred, the diagnosis no longer pertains to the resident's current status and does not need to be coded in item I3.

Downstaging ulcers

CMS requires staff to downstage ulcers as they heal for the purpose of MDS coding only. Although this practice goes against the National Pressure Ulcer Advisory Panel's recommendations, downstaging the ulcer for the MDS allows staff to track the healing progress of the wound. Stage the ulcer in regards to its appearance, according to the revised *RAI User's Manual*. For example, if a stage 3 pressure ulcer has healed so that it now resembles a stage 2, code the ulcer as a stage 2 in item M1 of the MDS.

Assessing risk

Assessment of the MDS items affecting the risk status for indicator 24 begins with the coding of transferring and bed mobility in section G—physical functioning and structural problems. Because you consider only the self-performance column for indicator 24, you should monitor the resident's overall ability to perform ADLs. As explained in quality indicators 8 and 17, you can obtain this self-performance score by reviewing the resident's status as reported by all shifts during the seven-day assessment period. ADL performance before this seven-day period should not be considered. Extensive assistance (a score of 3) and total dependence (a score of 4) for either bed mobility or transferring will flag high-risk status. The MDS form identifies the amount of assistance that qualifies as a score of 3 or 4. Once again, it is important to thoroughly read and understand these descriptors, in addition to questioning staff members on all shifts, reviewing the medical record documentation, and consulting with the resident and family members to determine the proper coding.

High-risk residents

The presence of a coma also places a resident in the high-risk category for pressure ulcer prevalence. Comatose (B1) is coded a 1 only if the resident has a documented diagnosis of either persistent vegetative state or coma.

End-stage disease (J5c), which is defined on the MDS as having 6 or fewer months to live, is the next item that places a resident in the high-risk category for indicator 24. The prediction of life expectancy is a judgment based on an observable deterioration of condition and supporting diagnosis. Caretakers should consult with physicians to determine whether box J5c should be checked for a particular resident.

The final item classifying a resident in the high-risk category is other current or more detailed diagnoses and ICD-9 codes (I3). As discussed previously, you should include current active diagnoses affecting the resident's health and behavioral status. Diagnoses affecting indicator 24 pertain to malnutrition. Some of the specific diagnoses included are nutritional edema (kwashiorkor), nutritional marasmus, and protein-calorie malnutrition. You should enter in item I3 of the MDS any of these diagnoses present in the medical record, which relate to current resident status. Once again, physician involvement and medical chart review can assist with this determination.

Low-risk residents

Residents who have a pressure ulcer and do not have one of the preceding high-risk factors are automatically placed in the low-risk category. As mentioned earlier in this chapter, pressure ulcers in low-risk residents are considered a serious sentinel event. Regulatory agencies will need to determine why residents who are not at risk for developing pressure ulcers are developing them. If a resident does not have difficulties with bed mobility or transferring, is not comatose or at the end stage of life, and is not malnourished, the prevalence of pressure ulcer development should be low or nonexistent.

Where do you stand?

If a facility has a high percentage of residents with pressure ulcers, or just one resident classified as low risk with a pressure ulcer, regulatory agencies will conduct further review to determine why these ulcers occurred. If a facility specializes in the care of residents with skin problems, this percentage is expected to be higher. If, however, it is determined that residents are developing pressure ulcers due to immobility or poor nutritional status, quality of care could be questioned.

At a Glance

Domain #11
Skin Care

Quality Indicators	MDS Items	MDS Codes
24. Prevalence of stage 1–4 pressure ulcers	M2a: Pressure ulcer	1, 2, 3, or 4, or;
	I3: Other current or more detailed diagnoses and ICD-9 codes	Diagnosis ICD-9 code is 707.0
High risk for QI #24	G1a Box A: Bed mobility self-performance	3 or 4, or;
	G1b Box A: Transfer self-performance	3 or 4
	OR	
	B1: Comatose	1, or;
	J5c: End-stage disease, 6 or fewer months to live	Box is checked, or;

Domain #8 (cont.)

Quality Indicators	MDS Items	MDS Codes
See previous page.	I3: Other current or more detailed diagnoses and ICD-9 codes	Diagnosis ICD-9 code is 260, 261, 262, 263.0, 263.1, 263.2, 263.8, or 263.9
Low risk for QI #24—All other residents not classified as high risk	N/A	N/A

Chapter 14

Reading and Interpreting Quality Indicator Reports

The MDS data, which are transmitted electronically, are used to determine which specific areas of nursing home care regulatory agencies should review and investigate. This raw MDS information is consolidated, interpreted, and displayed on six different report formats, available to both state regulatory agencies and nursing facilities at the MDS transmission computer site. The names of these reports are the following:

1. Facility quality indicator profile
2. Facility characteristics
3. Resident level quality indicator summary
4. Resident listing
5. Data submission summary
6. Assessment summary

Each of these reports contains valuable information designed to assist nursing facilities in pinpointing areas for continued quality improvement. To effectively use this data to improve resident care, facilities need to completely understand and correctly interpret each report.

Facility quality indicator profile

Which indicators have flagged?

The facility quality indicator profile probably contains the most important data; it shows which quality indicators have flagged. The profile lists the domains with the corresponding quality indicators, followed by columns of numerical data obtained from the MDS. The first column—number in numerator—lists the number of residents in the facility who have the quality indicator. The second column—number in denominator—lists the number of residents who have the potential for developing the quality indicator. In several quality indicators, certain conditions that prevent the indicator from occurring exclude specific residents. Therefore, the number in this column will not always be equal to the total number of residents in the facility who have a completed and transmitted MDS. The third column—facility percentage—is determined by dividing the numerator by the denominator and multiplying by 100.

Using facility percentage to determine where you stand

The facility percentage does not determine whether an indicator will flag because each facility must have a reference point to compare against. The comparison group percentage, the percentage of occurrence of each indicator for a set group of facilities, is compared with the individual nursing home to obtain the percentile ranking. A high percentile ranking means the nursing facility has a higher percentage of residents with the presence of the quality indicator than the comparison group; a low ranking means the facility has a lower percentage of residents with the presence of the indicator than the comparison group.

Identifying and fixing your weak areas

A small picture of a flag indicates high percentile rankings. A flag marks either an indicator at or greater than the ninetieth percentile rank or the presence of a sentinel event. Although a sentinel event might not raise that quality indicator up to the ninetieth percentile, one resident with the event will cause the indicator to flag.

Therefore, because the flagged indicators denote an area affecting more residents than expected, investigators must determine why so many residents are included. As discussed at the conclusion of each quality indicator, a facility might specialize in the care of residents who flag an indicator; this does not necessarily mean there is a lack of quality care at the facility. However, if the problem is due to improper care and procedures, regulatory sanctions could be imposed.

Report settings

When obtaining the facility quality indicator report, you can choose a variety of settings to individualize the data for the desired information. The default settings, or quick settings, report MDS data from a six-month period ending with the final day of the last full calendar month. The comparison group is all state facilities for a designated three-month period. The available custom settings can change the report period to any desired time frame. If a facility wishes to compare the usual six-month period with a shorter time period to observe whether more or fewer quality indicators are flagged, it can change the time frame's beginning date and ending date. If MDS training and inservice courses were recently provided, comparing two different time periods of data might provide information about the effectiveness of the training, as evidenced by more accurate coding of the MDS form.

In the custom setting, the comparison group time period can also be selected. A three-month period of the facility's choosing can be used for comparison group purposes. This option is useful when changing the dates of the reporting period. For example, if a facility wishes to obtain the quality indicator report for data from a period before the quick settings period, it can choose the data from the comparison group to reflect that same time period.

Facility percentage at a glance: Using graphs to analyze your raw data

A graphical representation of a facility's percentage as it relates to the comparison group percentage can be a valuable tool for long-term care (LTC) administrators (Figure 14.1). Assuming that default report settings are used and that the comparison group state percentage for a six-month period for quality indicator 2—prevalence of falls—remained the same at 15%, you can easily compare this number to the facility percentage for falls. During the first time period, this sample facility had a 26% prevalence of falls; however, after five months, this number dropped to 10%. You can easily illustrate internal progress in decreasing the number of falls. If no progress is shown, planning for quality improvement could be implemented.

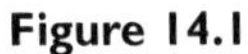

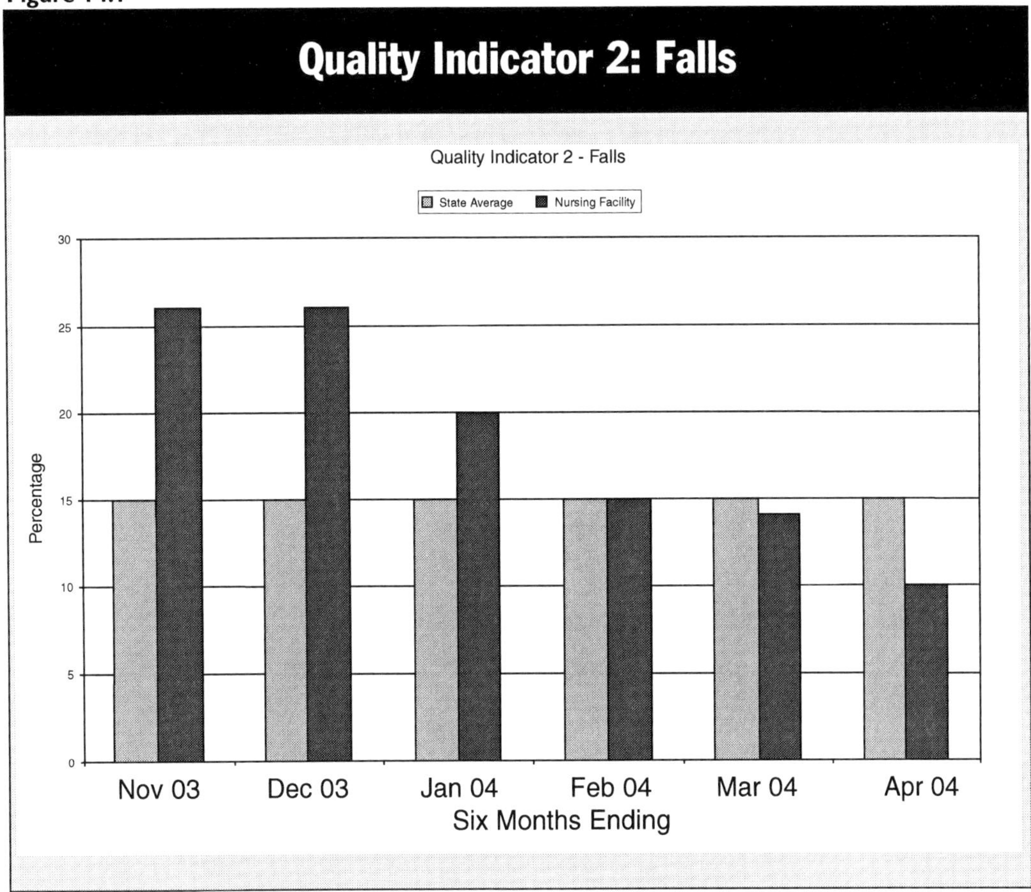

Facility characteristics

Demographic information

The facility characteristics report includes demographic information that will help determine possible reasons for the flagging of quality indicators. This report includes information about resident gender, age, payment source, diagnosis, assessment types, stability of conditions, and statistics regarding discharge potential. The first column—number of residents—identifies how many residents in the facility are placed in each of the categories. The facility percentage is determined by calculating the number of residents that have each characteristic with the total number of residents. Once again, the report provides a comparison group percentage to compare how the individual facility findings relate to a larger set of nursing facilities. This report does not include a percentile ranking or flagging.

Number of residents in each category

If a category has either a high or low number of residents compared to the larger group of facilities, this helps to explain the presence of a quality indicator. For example, if a facility codes many residents as having an end-stage disease, it might be expected that the prevalence of bedfast residents is higher than the comparison group. If a facility codes many residents as having a potential for discharge, the number of bedfast residents might be lower. The information from this report only assists in explaining the reasons for quality indicator flagging; finding the cause requires more investigation.

Report settings

As with the quality indicator profile report, the facility characteristics report can be obtained using quick settings or can be individualized with custom settings. The quick settings option uses MDS data from the six-month period ending with the last full calendar month and compares this data with all state facilities for a specified three-month period. Custom settings can change the beginning and ending date of the MDS data for the report period and the three-month period of comparison group data.

Resident level quality indicator summary

Once the facility quality indicator profile is obtained, learn which specific residents are included in the numerator for each quality indicator. The resident level quality indicator summary provides this information. The summary lists each resident, along with the most recent MDS date, and reason for the MDS assessment. Each quality indicator, including high- and low-risk adjustments for four quality indicators, is listed in columns. A check mark indicates that the resident's MDS was coded to reflect that specific indicator. If a resident was discharged during the report time period, this information is also specified. Finally, the number of quality indicator check marks for each resident is added and presented in the total column. The numerical value for the total column can range from 0 (no quality indicator present) to 28 (all indicators plus risk adjustments present).

The specified number of residents in the numerator of the quality indicator report will be either identical to or less than the number of residents identified with that quality indicator on the resident level quality indicator summary. The facility quality indicator profile does not include data from the initial admission assessment, whereas the resident level quality indicator summary includes data from all MDS forms, including the admission assessment. Therefore, the facility quality indicator profile does not include those residents on the resident level summary report who are listed as a "01" in assessment reason AA8a.

When interpreting this resident level quality indicator summary, primarily review those quality indicators that flagged and the residents designated as having the indicator present. Also review the total column; those residents who have a high number of quality indicators have the potential for care issues, and the reasons for this high number must be determined. Once again, a facility might specialize in the care of extremely medically complex residents, which could result in a high number of residents with quality indicators present.

Report settings

Use either quick or custom settings when obtaining the resident level quality indicator summary. The quick settings option uses the six-month period of MDS data, ending with the most recent full calendar month. This report includes all residents with a completed MDS form with any coded reason for the assessment. The custom settings option allows the time frame for the MDS data report period to be changed to individualize the report to meet the facility's needs. Additionally, a custom settings choice is available that only lists those residents who flagged one or more quality indicators. Residents who have a score of 0 in the total column (no quality indicators present) are not listed. This report does not use a comparison group; therefore, a custom option is not available for this area.

Resident listing

The resident listing is a summary report of all residents with MDS forms submitted during the designated report period. This report lists the resident identification as coded on the MDS, resident name, most recent and previous assessment dates and reasons, discharge date (if applicable), room number, date of birth, Social Security number, and Medicare number. The report can be used to easily determine which MDS form for each resident is providing the information affecting the quality indicator. For the four quality indicators considered incidence indicators, this report also identifies the two MDS forms being compared (the most recent and previous assessments) that measure changes in resident status over time. Therefore, the residents with incidence indicators can be identified from the resident level quality indicator summary, and the MDS forms used for determining the incidence can be verified with the resident listing. Similar to the resident quality indicator summary, the resident listing indicates who has been discharged during the report period and shows the actual discharge date.

Report settings

The quick settings option automatically includes MDS data from a six-month period, ending with the most recent full calendar month. Choosing custom settings changes the beginning and ending dates of the report time frame to the facility's preference. If you change the facility quality indicator profile and resident quality indicator summary reports to a custom-report time period, changing this report to that same time period allows for accurate comparison of data.

Data submission summary

The data submission summary includes information related to the number of MDS forms transmitted during a specific time frame. The assessments submitted are grouped by month of submission date and include the production submissions, or number of times that MDS forms were transmitted during a specific month. The unique residents column identifies the number of residents for which MDSs were received, and the total assessments accepted indicates how many MDSs were transmitted during a one-month time period. Finally, the total assessments accepted are categorized according to the reason for the MDS assessment in the accepted assessments by type category.

Because it is necessary for MDS forms to be submitted at least every 31 days, this report is an excellent tool to determine whether this requirement is being met. If a calendar month does not have a production submission, investigate to see whether the MDS forms are still being submitted in a timely manner.

Report settings

The quick settings option results in the report period being five full calendar months and the current month from the first day to the day before the day the reports are being requested. Therefore, the information on this report is updated more frequently than monthly, and you can access a report with new information after each production submission. This report routinely has up to six months of data.

The custom settings option allows two changes of settings. The report period can be changed from the preset period to a time period preferred by the facility by changing the beginning and ending dates of the period. Additionally, the facility can change the number of months included in the body of the report to reflect more or fewer months before the report request date than the quick settings option of six months. If a facility wishes to view its MDS submission information for a longer or shorter period, this option is available.

Assessment summary

The assessment summary lists the MDS forms submitted by month of assessment reference date. Whereas the previous report considers the day the MDS was transmitted, this report considers the day the MDS was submitted by identifying the MDS assessment reference date. This report does not include production submissions, but it does include the number of residents with a submitted MDS and the total assessments completed by month according to the assessment reference date. Once again, this report classifies the accepted assessments according to the reason for the MDS completion. This is a good tool to use when determining whether the MDS forms are being completed on a regular basis. If a month has a low number of unique residents, either the facility was not completing MDS forms on time or fewer MDS forms were required during that month.

Report settings

Both the quick settings and custom settings for this report are similar to the previous report. Quick settings display five full calendar months and the current month up to the day before the report request. Up to six months of data make up the body of the report.

Custom settings allow the facility to change the beginning and ending dates of the report period to reflect the time period the facility chooses. Once again, the number of months for which data is provided can also be increased or decreased from the customary six-month time period to reflect individual facility needs. This change either decreases or increases the number of months shown going back from the report request date.

Using the reports effectively

Because all the information from these six reports is available to regulatory agencies, it is crucial that nursing facilities obtain these reports and review them carefully. Nursing facilities should set up a routine schedule for downloading this information, and all appropriate personnel should be involved in the interpretation and discussion of the data. Only by thoroughly reading and understanding the large amount of available information can LTC facilities determine which quality indicators need further investigation and whether quality of care is present.

How surveyors choose their focus

When it comes to actual survey time, it shouldn't be a secret as to which residents the surveyors are going to examine closely. When they enter the building, they will already have accessed your quality indicator reports, which tell them what indicators put your facility in the 75th percentile or higher. That means that you have a higher incidence or prevalence in a quality indicator than 74% of the nation's nursing homes. Here's how surveyors use the quality indicators when they inspect a facility for its annual survey:

- For a 120-bed facility, surveyors will probably choose 20–25 residents' records to scrutinize. Five of those residents will undergo a **comprehensive review,** which means that surveyors will examine the indicators related to these residents that show up on the quality indicator report.

- The other 15–20 are subject to **focused reviews,** based on concerns surveyors dig up prior to the inspection.

- You can also expect surveyors to conduct about three reviews of residents with **closed records**—residents who transferred to other facilities, went home, or passed away. These will include residents involved in complaint investigations.
- Finally, surveyors are sure to review any residents' records involving **sentinel events,** which include the previously mentioned indicators of dehydration, pressure ulcers, plus any incidents of fecal impaction.

Surveyors will electronically receive these quality indicator reports on a particular facility close to the survey date, so that they use the latest MDS data. You can request quality indicator reports for your own facility at any time, but you should check them frequently during your survey window. This will allow you to gauge which residents surveyors will spotlight during survey.

Chapter 15

The Quality Measures

The quality measures, similar to the quality indicators, are an attempt by the Center for Medicare & Medicaid Services (CMS) not only to define quality care but also to measure objectively quality in specific areas of long-term care delivery by using data from the MDS assessment form. These measures are made available to the public on the Internet. Prospective residents and their families can access quality measure percentages for your facility that, in theory, represent whether quality care is provided there.

It is important to protect your facility's reputation for providing quality care. If staff, families, and residents don't understand what the quality measures are all about, your facility could be unfairly categorized as a poor-performing provider. Therefore, access your quality measures on the Web by going to *www.medicare.gov/NHCompare* to keep yourself updated on your scores. Additionally, teach your staff about the quality measures and explain percentages to families and residents.

Birth of the quality measures

The quality measures began as a part of the Nursing Home Quality Initiative led by CMS. In early 2002, CMS started a pilot project in six states—Colorado, Florida, Maryland, Ohio, Rhode Island, and Washington. Two of the major objectives are to determine whether the original quality measures were indeed effective in defining quality and to provide this information to consumers of nursing home services.

The quality measures program started nationwide in the fall of 2002 after the conclusion of the pilot study. Based on information provided by the pilot study, CMS deleted some measures and changed others to make them more accurate measures of quality care. CMS came out with a revised set of quality measures about a year later and continues to refine them today.

Several of the most important decisions made after the pilot study related to whether the quality measures were reliable and valid. CMS believed that it must measure quality consistently across a variety of settings and that it must measure quality of care as it related to good resident outcomes. Additionally, CMS required that the information reported to the public be information consumers would actually use when choosing a nursing home or when questioning the care provided at a facility.

Two types of measures

The quality measures chosen relate to two different types of nursing home resident populations: chronic care and postacute care. Chronic care residents are typically long-term residents admitted because they are unable to care for themselves. These residents remain in the nursing home for a long period of time or permanently, with no discharge anticipated.

Postacute care residents, however, stay at a facility for a shorter period of time, frequently no longer than 30 days. These residents are usually admitted following a hospital stay and require intense nursing or rehabilitative services prior to returning home.

Tackling the quality measures

Many skilled nursing facility leaders are falling behind in that they haven't studied all the nuances of the enhanced quality measures. Similarly, nursing home providers may be more familiar with the original set of measures, released in November 2002.

Additionally, providers don't tend to log on to the Web site that they use for MDS transmission to get the latest quality measure scores and information—but they should. Even if they are aware of the measures, that information isn't always getting to frontline staff, who are instrumental in causing change. The administrator therefore needs to get the word out and raise awareness to effect positive change.

Such efforts are especially necessary now that the public is using the Nursing Home Compare Web site more frequently—consumers will want to know why certain measures of your facility are higher (i.e., appear worse) than the local or national averages. In 2003, 9.3 million people visited the Nursing Home Compare Web site, and 5.9 million people used its call center. That number is expected to continue to grow.

Because quality measures can create a lasting first impression for a potential resident or family member who logs on to Nursing Home Compare to look up your scores, use the following four tips to keep your measures on the up-and-up.

Banish ignorance

Management needs to get in the habit of tracking the facility's scores so they know what the measures say about the facility. Check your computer regularly for updates, as the quality measures will post on a quarterly basis in the electronic mailbox that you use for MDS transmission. Keep in touch with your state's quality improvement organization—the organization CMS charged with helping nursing homes improve their quality measures scores —and try your own association's Web site for updates.

Remember that quality measures aren't just for the public. They're for nursing homes to observe their own progress in improving care. If you keep on top of your scores and know what they mean, you can catch issues before they become downward trends in care. Of course, nursing homes can do everything in their power to provide good care and still have skewed numbers for one measure or another, but if they know how the measures are figured, they can determine why their numbers look wrong.

Embrace MDS accuracy initiatives

When evaluating your data, the first area to review is the source of the quality measure information—the MDS. The staff member who completes this assessment tool must have the training and knowledge to prepare it correctly. Make sure that this individual attends regular training sessions and keeps up with the many updates and changes to MDS coding rules.

Don't make the mistake of simply chasing improved scores—on quality measures or quality indicators—and think that it will solve all your assessment improvement and quality care issues. If you see that a score is inordinately high compared with that of other facilities, it may be an

MDS accuracy issue rather than a care issue. Dig deeper into finding out what caused the score, rather than just initiating numerous efforts to bring down the score right away.

Boost resident care systems

If you have a quality measure problem that's not the result of incorrect MDS coding, then you can turn to your care practices and see what could improve in that area. For instance, there has always been a quality measure for pain because studies indicate that it's a resident care process that facilities could improve almost universally.

To start improving this process, facilities should kill the concept of prn, or medications for residents with continuous pain. Residents are often in significant pain by the time a prn medication kicks in, so facilities should try a reverse prn method instead. That means administering the medication routinely unless residents specifically say they don't want it.

For residents with fairly continuous pain, prn medications should be used for breakthrough pain only. Look up clinical practice guidelines, such as those from the American Medical Directors Association, for further help with pain assessment and management.

Monitor outcomes

It's not enough to put new systems in place that you think could improve resident outcomes—you have to monitor them as well. For instance, facilities that become better at tracking pain might experience an increase in the number of residents who report feeling pain for a short time following improvement efforts. That's because staff became better at recognizing and reporting resident pain—not because more residents are in pain. Eventually, the number of residents who trigger the pain quality measure should decrease as your treatment methods improve.

Responding to residents and families

Be sure to explain the quality measures to residents, family members, and future customers of your nursing home in a language they can understand. If your quality measures uncover a negative care issue, be ready to discuss initiatives your facility has already put in place to deal with the problem.

Consumers typically will express the most concern about a quality measure percentage that seems to be higher than other nursing homes. To handle such concerns, learn how each quality measure is calculated and be able to convey that information to families and residents. Provide an explanation for any percentages that seem extreme, and be prepared to discuss any quality improvement programs your facility is using to improve care in any needed area. Also, if the quality measure data is inaccurate, explain why.

Chapter 16

Ensuring Quality Care

The quality indicators: A road map for optimum care

The 24 quality indicators serve as a guide to determine whether quality care is present. However, if a particular indicator does not flag, that does not necessarily guarantee that quality care is being provided in that area. Therefore, nursing facilities should not only monitor quality indicator reports but also consider internal quality improvement activities.

How can you ensure quality in your facility? Making sure that you meet regulatory requirements for each of the quality indicators should start you off in the right direction. Instead of simply meeting basic required standards, nursing facilities should seek to exceed and improve on CMS' quality standards. The quality indicators are a guideline to help facilities focus on potential areas for quality improvement actions. However, facilities should not stop there. For example, if the prevalence of daily physical restraints is below the percentile rank that would cause concern, but is still too high in the facility's judgment, the facility should establish restraint reduction programs. Using the MDS data to direct their efforts, staff can investigate whether any one section of the nursing home uses more restraints than other sections, whether the restraints are used more on certain shifts, or whether specific staff members apply restraints more freely than other staff members. As the staff conducts further investigation of each of these areas, they may hone in on potential solutions or the implementation of systems that may continue to decrease restraint use. Eliciting ideas from all staff members, especially nursing assistants who typically have the most direct contact with the residents, can yield excellent recommendations for improvement in all the quality domains.

Tools on the Web

Ensure that your quality indicators are correct by making sure you are coding the MDS accurately. CMS comes out with periodic updates to its revised *Resident Assessment Instrument User's Manual*, which you should utilize as soon as they are released. Access these changes in either of the two following ways:

- Go to *www.hcpro.com/long-term-care* and scroll down to the Long-Term Care Resource Center at the bottom of the page. Click on "MDS/PPS" and scroll down on that page to the "Government Documents" section in blue. There you will find listed all the updated to the *Resident Assessment Instrument User's Manual* since it was revised in 2003. You will also have access to the latest MDS and PPS news from the same Web site.

- Go to *www.cms.hhs.gov/quality/mds20* to download the revised *Resident Assessment Instrument User's Manual* and its updates.

- Go to *www.medicare.gov/NHCompare/home.asp* to look up your quality measure scores and the recent deficiencies you acquired in your survey.

Consumers may also use this Web site to access your quality data and compare your facility's performance with that of others.

The importance of proactive care planning

Accurate assessment and completion of the MDS are only two aspects of continual quality care. The quality indicator information obtained from the MDS assessments begins the process for determining quality, but it cannot end there. Based on careful scrutiny of the assessment data and quality indicators which have flagged, facilities must make appropriate plans to maintain or improve quality issues and implement them. Actual ideas and methods determined to be important and beneficial need to be put in place. Finally, evaluation of the effectiveness of the action or plan should reveal the need for revisions or adjustments.

The 24 quality indicators provide a starting point for defining and measuring what it means to deliver quality care to our residents. However, they only provide one piece of the puzzle. In the final analysis, what constitutes "quality" care is a highly personal and subjective matter and depends on the individuals involved. The quality indicators can point a long-term care (LTC) center in the proper direction and provide the framework for proper care planning. However, the continual planning, implementation, and evaluation process should be individualized for each facility, based on the particular needs of the residents. A quality improvement plan that works extremely well in one nursing center might be completely wrong for another nursing center. Each facility should determine its own strengths and weaknesses and implement plans for quality improvement through an in-depth analysis of its unique quality concerns.

Although these 24 quality indicators were designed as a tool to more objectively measure quality, undoubtedly changes and additions to this system will arise. Will an ideal, comprehensive system guaranteed to completely measure quality ever be developed? Probably not. Quality is a subjective concept meaning different things for different people. Although one resident at a LTC center may be pleased with the level of service provided, the resident in the next room might perceive a lack of quality, although they receive identical services. Healthcare providers should consider all of the varying perceptions and ideas about quality and attempt to provide both required and requested healthcare services for all residents.

Most caretakers entered the healthcare field because they wanted to take good care of people and promote health. Similarly, providing optimum care for residents is the main goal of every long-term facility. Quality is an abstract concept; but this healthcare mission—to provide the best possible care—is the common theme. Maintaining and promoting the dignity and independence of every elderly resident are paramount to achieving this goal. Through dedication to the commitment of ensuring quality care, the healthcare industry can use the information from the quality indicators to rise to an even higher level of success in patient care.

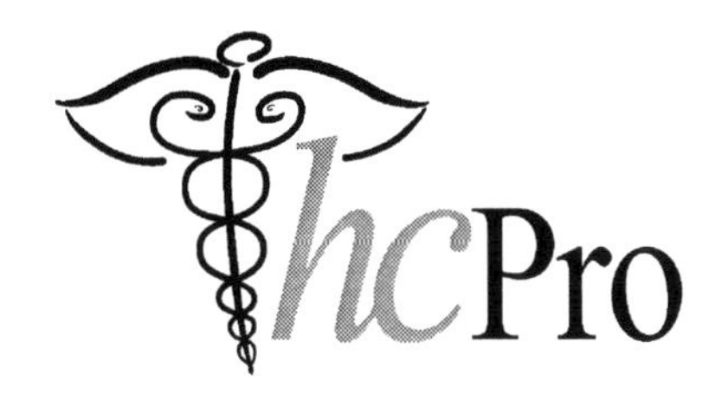

Related Products from HCPro

Books

- *60 Essential Forms for Long-Term Care Documentation*
- *Collections 1, 2, 3: Proven Strategies for Collecting Long-Term Care Accounts Receivable*
- *Defensive Documentation for Long-Term Care: Strategies for Creating a More Lawsuit-Proof Resident Record*
- *Long-Term Care Risk Management: Pressure Ulcers*
- *Long-Term Care Risk Management: Resident Falls*
- *MDS Troubleshooter, Second Edition*
- *Survey Troubleshooter: Proven Strategies for Mastering the Top 25 Nursing Home Deficiencies*

Newsletters

- *PPS Alert for Long-Term Care*
- *Billing Alert for Long-Term Care*
- *Briefings on Long-Term Care Regulations*

To obtain additional information, to order any of the aforementioned products, or to comment on *Quality Indicators, Second Edition: A Practical Guide to Assessment and Documentation*, please contact us at:

HCPro, Inc.
P.O. Box 1168
Marblehead, MA 01945
Toll-free telephone: 800/650-6787
Toll-free fax: 800/639-8511
E-mail: *customerservice@hcpro.com*
Internet: *www.hcmarketplace.com*